THE ANATOMY
OF THE
HUMAN PERITONEUM
AND
ABDOMINAL CAVITY

BY
GEORGE S. HUNTINGTON

PREFACE.

In the following pages an attempt has been made to emphasize the value of Embryology and Comparative Anatomy in elucidating the difficult and often complicated morphological problems encountered in the study of human adult anatomy.

Moreover, in addition to the direct advance in the method and scope of anatomical teaching afforded by these aids, it is further hoped that the broader interpretation, both of structure and function, obtained by ontogenetic and phylogenetic comparison, will impart an interest to the study of adult human morphology, such as the subject, considered solely in the narrow field of its own limitations, could never arouse.

The book represents part of the course in visceral anatomy as developed during the past fourteen years at Columbia University. The sections dealing with the morphology of the vertebrate ileo-colic junction and with the structural details of the human cæcum and appendix are considered somewhat more fully, as warranted by the extensive material available. The illustrations are for the greater part taken from preparations in the Morphological Museum of the University. Wherever practicable the direct photographic reproduction of the actual preparation is given. In the case of preparations not suitable for this purpose, careful drawings have been made which offer in every instance a faithful and correct interpretation of the conditions presented by the actual object. A number of the embryonic illustrations are taken from the standard text-books on the subject, due credit being given to their source. I desire to express my sincere thanks to Dr. Edward Leaming, of the Department of Photography and to Mr. M. Petersen, artist of the Anatomical Department of the University, for their skilful and thoroughly reliable work in the preparation of the illustrations.

GEORGE S. HUNTINGTON.

COLUMBIA   UNIVERSITY,   in   the   City   of   New   York, *December, 1902.*

INTRODUCTION.

In considering the anatomy of the human abdominal cavity and peritoneum in the following pages the explanation of the adult conditions encountered is based upon the development of the parts, and the successive human embryonal stages are illustrated by the examination of the lower vertebrates presenting permanent adult structural conditions which appear as merely temporary embryonal stages in the development of the higher mammalian alimentary tract.

For the sake of clearness and brevity all discussion of the *theories of peritoneal development* has been designedly omitted. The assumption of peritoneal *adhesion*, and consequent obliteration of serous areas, offers many advantages in considering the adult human abdominal cavity, especially from the standpoint of comparative anatomy. The same has consequently been adopted without reference to divergent views and theories.

In studying the descriptive text and the diagrams the student should remember that the volume offers in no sense a complete or detailed account of the development of the abdominal cavity and its contents. The purpose is not to present the embryology of this portion of the vertebrate body, but to *utilize* certain embryological facts in order to *explain* the complicated adult conditions encountered. To avoid confusion, and to bring the salient points into strong relief, the majority of the diagrams illustrating human embryonal stages are purely schematic.

Moreover, in order to avoid confusing and unnecessary details it is often desirable to disregard developmental chronology entirely. Many of the diagrams combine several successive developmental stages, showing different degrees of development in different portions of the same drawing. Again it is frequently necessary, for the sake of brevity and clearness, to actually depart from known embryological conditions. If, for example, the stomach and liver are treated as if they were from their inception abdominal organs, the student of systematic embryology will recall the fact that this position is only *obtained after* their primitive differentiation by growth and migration.

Again the mesenteries are treated here as if they formed definite and well-defined membranes from the beginning—without reference to the abdominal organs with which they are associated. We speak of the liver as growing into and between the layers of the ventral mesogastrium, because this conception offers the opportunity of more clearly explaining the adult condition. Actually, however, the membrane develops, as a new structure, after the first differentiation of liver and stomach, as these organs descend into the abdominal cavity.

Similar discrepancies between fact and schema are encountered throughout. Consequently, while the purpose of the volume is to facilitate the study and comprehension of the *adult*peritoneal cavity and its contents, the reader should guard against receiving the developmental illustration as a correct successive and detailed account of the *embryology* of the parts concerned.

In like manner the comparative anatomical facts adduced form in no sense even approximately a complete serial morphological account of the vertebrate alimentary tract.

To the student of human anatomy the zoölogical position of the forms which help him to understand complicated human structural conditions is immaterial. He can draw on all the vertebrate classes independently of their mutual relations. Hence neither ontogeny nor phylogeny are here introduced, except as aids to the study of adult human anatomy. The following pages offer neither an embryology nor a comparative anatomy of the alimentary tract, but an attempt has been made in them to illustrate the significance of the complicated anatomical details presented by the adult human abdominal cavity by reference to the simpler antecedent conditions encountered during the early developmental stages of the higher forms and permanently in the structure of the lower vertebrates.

While, as just stated, a complete presentation of the development of the abdominal cavity is not required, yet the student will find it of advantage to rehearse the main facts of vertebrate embryology, for the purpose of bringing a clear understanding of the manner in which the vertebrate body is built up to bear upon the problems which the special organs and structures of the body-cavity present for his consideration. This purpose can be accomplished by a very brief and condensed consideration of the cardinal facts.

FIG. 1.—Human ovum, from a mature follicle, a sphere of about 0.2 mm. diameter. × 25. (Kollmann.)

FIG. 2.—Segmentation of mammalian ovum (bat). (After E. von Beneden.) Two blastomeres, each with a nucleus, shown in lighter color. The dark bodies are yolk-granules.

FIG. 3.—Segmentation of mammalian ovum. Four blastomeres. (After E. von Beneden.)

The entire vertebrate body is the product of developmental changes taking place after fertilization in a single primitiveCELL, the EGG or OVUM (Fig. 1).

In structure the ovum corresponds to other animal cells. On account of their special significance during development the different component parts of the egg-cell have received special distinctive names. The *cell-body*is known as the *vitellus* or *yolk*. It is composed of two substances, the *protoplasm* or formative yolk and the *deuteroplasm* or nutritive yolk, which vary in their relative proportions in the ova of different animals.

The protoplasm represents the material from which in the course of development the cells forming the body of the individual are derived, while the deuteroplasm serves for the nutrition of the ovum during the earliest stages of development.

The *nucleus* of the egg-cell is distinguished as the *germinal vesicle*, and its *nucleolus* as the*germinal spot*.

The *cell-body* or *vitellus* is surrounded by a condensed portion of the cell contents to which the name of the vitelline membrane has been applied, which in turn is enclosed by a transparent and elastic cover, the*zona pellucida*, presenting a radially striated appearance.

The ovum is contained in the cortical portion of the ovary, enclosed in the *Graafian follicle*, a vesicle 4-8 mm. in diameter, whose fibrous walls are lined by several layers of epithelial cells, which surround the ovum, forming the *discus proligerus*.

After impregnation the egg-cell, by a process of repeated division or cleavage, undergoes*segmentation*, the cell-body being divided successively into two, four, eight, sixteen,

2

thirty-two, etc., *cells*, called *blastomeres* (Figs. 2 and 3). The mass of cells finally resulting from this process of segmentation forms the ground work of the future body. A vertebrate ovum in this stage of complete segmentation is called the *morula* from its resemblance to a mulberry (Fig. 4).

After segmentation is completed a cavity filled with fluid and surrounded by the developing cells is gradually formed in the interior of the mass. This cavity is known as the *segmentation-cavity*. The egg is now called the *blastula, blastosphere* or *blastodermic vesicle* and the cellular membrane enclosing the segmentation-cavity forms the *germinal membrane* or *blastoderm* (Figs. 5 and 6). The cells of the blastoderm become aggregated at one point on the circumference of the vesicle (dorsal pole of blastosphere) forming, when viewed from above, a thickened biscuit or disk-shaped opaque area. This is known as the *germinal area*, or *primitive blastoderm* or *embryonic shield* (Figs. 7 and 12).

FIG. 4.—Ovum of rabbit, from terminal portion of oviduct. The zona pellucida appears thickened, and contains many spermatozoa which failed to penetrate the ovum. (After Bischoff.)

FIG. 5.—Blastodermic vesicle of rabbit. (After E. von Beneden.)

FIG. 6.—Blastodermic vesicle of *Triton tæniatus*. (Hertwig.)

FIG. 7.—Embryonic area of rabbit embryo. (Heisler, after E. von Beneden.) The primitive streak beginning in the cell-proliferation known as the "node of Hensen."

This is the first indication of the coming division of the entire egg-cell into the *embryo proper* and the *vitelline* or *yolk-sac* (Figs. 8 and 9). The entire future individual develops from the cells of the germinal area. This area comprises both the embryo proper and the region immediately surrounding it.

FIG. 8.—Blastodermic vesicle of mammal. (E. von Beneden.) The layer of cells lining the interior of the vesicle next to the zona pellucida forms Rauber's "Deckschichte" or prochorion. This is not the true ectoderm, since it does not participate in the formation of the embryo, which is entirely derived from the cells of the germinal area.

FIG. 9.—Human embryo with yolk-sac, amnion, and belly-stalk of fifteen to eighteen days. (Heisler, after Coste.)

The remainder of the ovum, serving temporary purposes of nutrition and respiration, gradually becomes absorbed and disappears.

FIG. 10.—Embryonal area of sheep, composed of ectoderm and entoderm. (After Bonnet.)

FIG. 11.—Blastodermic vesicle of rabbit. Section through embryonic area at caudal limit of node of Hensen. (Rabl.)

Transverse sections at right angles to the long axis of the embryonic area show that the single layer of cells composing the primitive germinal membrane becomes differentiated first into two (Fig. 10) and subsequently into three layers of cells (Fig. 11). At the margins of the germinal area these layers are of course continuous with the rest of yolk-sac wall. From their position in reference to the center of the cell the three layers of the blastoderm are described as—

1. The outer, Epiblast or Ectoderm.
2. The middle, Mesoblast or Mesoderm.
3. The inner, Hypoblast or Entoderm.

The central nervous system (brain and spinal cord) is derived from the ectoderm by the development of a groove in the long axis of the embryonic area (Figs. 13, 14, 16 and 17), and by the subsequent union in the dorsal midline of the ridges bounding the groove to form a closed tube (Fig. 18). (Medullary groove, plates and canal.)

FIG. 12.—Oval embryonic area of rabbit's egg, detached with part of wall of

FIG. 13.—Transverse section of embryonic area of ovum of sheep of fourteen and a half days. (Heisler, after Bonnet.)

3

blastodermic vesicle. × 30. (Kollmann.)

FIG. 14.—Germinal area of rabbit's ovum. (Kollmann.)

FIG. 15.—Surface-view of area pellucida of an eighteen-hour chick-embryo. (Balfour.)

FIG. 16.—Transverse section of human embryo before development of protovertebræ or chorda dorsalis. (Keibel.)

FIG. 17.—Transverse section of a sixteen and a half day sheep embryo. (Heisler, after Bonnet.)

FIG. 18.—Embryo of bird, at beginning of third day, with four blastodermic layers, resulting from the division of the mesoderm into parietal and visceral layers, separated by the cœlom cavity. Transverse section. × 170. (Kollmann.)

The following changes in the ventral aspect lead to the formation of the alimentary canal and body-cavity:

The developing embryo at first lies flat on the subjacent yolk-mass, and subsequently becomes gradually separated more and more from the rest of the blastoderm by grooves or furrows which develop along the sides and at the cephalic and caudal extremity of the embryo. The folds resulting from these furrows indent the yolk more and more as development proceeds and tend to approach each other at a central point, the future *umbilicus*.

In the meanwhile changes in the region of the mesoderm have led to conditions which produce a differentiation of the ventral portion of the embryo into two tubes or cylinders, the *alimentary* or *intestinal canal* and the *general body-cavity*, the former being included within the latter.

Early in the course of development a number of spaces appear in the mesoderm on each side of the axial line of the embryo. These spaces soon unite to form two large cavities, one on each side. Taken together these cavities constitute the *cœlom* or *body-cavity*, which becomes subdivided in the adult mammal into the pleural, pericardial and abdominal cavities.

As these cœlom cavities develop in the mesoderm the cells lining them become distinctly epithelial. This mesodermic epithelium lining the cœlom is called the *mesothelium*.

The development of the cœlom space divides the mesoderm on each side into an outer leaf, the *somatic* or *parietal mesoderm*, and an inner leaf, the *splanchnic* or *visceral mesoderm* (Figs. 18 and 19). The former is closely applied to the ectoderm, forming with it the *somatopleure* or *body-wall*. The latter, in close contact with the entoderm, forms with it the *splanchnopleure* or wall of the alimentary canal. In the dorsal median line both somatic and splanchnic mesoderm become continuous with each other and with the axial mesoderm (Fig. 20).

FIG. 19.—Transverse section of a seventeen and a half day sheep embryo. (Bonnet.)

FIG. 20.—Curves of blastodermic layers and division of mesoderm in amniote embryo. (Kollmann.)

The folds of the splanchnopleure, indenting the yolk-sac, form a gutter directly connected with the yolk, the *primitive intestinal groove* or *furrow*, whose margins gradually approach each other (Fig. 20). In this way the primitive alimentary canal becomes separated from the yolk. At first this separation is ill-defined, and the channel of communication between the primitive intestine and the yolk is wide (Figs. 13,16, 17 and 19). The folding of the splanchnopleure completes, at an early period, the dorsal and lateral walls of the embryonic gut, but ventrally, toward the yolk, the tube is incomplete and widely open.

By union and coalescence of the splanchnopleural folds, proceeding from the caudal and cephalic ends towards the center, this primitive wide channel gradually becomes narrowed down, until the communication between the yolk-sac and the intestine is reduced to a canal, the *vitello-intestinal* or *omphalo-mesenteric duct*. The intestinal gutter is thus converted into a closed tube except at the point of implantation of the vitelline duct during the persistence of this structure. In the meanwhile the somatopleural folds forming the body-walls grow more and more together from the sides, approaching the vitello-intestinal duct. Finally touching each other they coalesce to form the ventral body wall, in the same manner as the splanch[n]opleural folds met and united to form the alimentary tube.

At the same time the vitello-intestinal duct and the remnant of the yolk-sac, to which it was attached ("umbilical vesicle"), normally become obliterated and disappear.

4

After the intestinal tube and the body cavity have thus become closed the embryo straightens out and the alimentary canal appears as a nearly straight cylindrical tube extending from the cephalic to the caudal end of the embryo. This primitive alimentary tube at first terminates at its cephalic extremity in a blind pouch, while at the caudal end in the early stages the intestine is connected with the nerve-tube by a channel called the *neuro-enteric canal*, forming in the earliest embryos a communication between the ectoderm lining the bottom of the medullary groove and the entoderm (Figs. 22 and 26). In man this stage is encountered very early, in embryos of 2 mm. before the formation of either heart or provertebræ.

FIG. 21.—Sagittal section of caudal extremity of cat embryo of 6 mm. (Tourneux.)

FIG. 22.—Caudal half of human blastoderm measuring 3 mm., with open medullary groove. Dorsal view. × 30. (After Spee.)

At the point where the canal develops the primitive groove presents a thickened circumvallate spot, marking the beginning perforation of the medullary plate from the ectoderm to the entoderm. The canal exists only for a short period during the earliest stages of embryonal life. It becomes rapidly closed, the neural and intestinal tubes henceforth remaining permanently separated from each other.

The embryonal caudal end of the primitive alimentary canal is not the final adult termination of the tube. When the anal aperture is formed in a manner to be presently detailed, the opening is situated cephalad of the portion connected with the nerve-tube by the neuro-enteric canal. Hence this terminal portion of the early embryonic alimentary canal is called the "post-anal gut" (Fig. 21).

The post-anal gut and the neuro-enteric canal are better developed in the embryos of the lower than in those of the higher vertebrates. But in all vertebrates of the present day both of these structures undergo regressive changes and finally disappear altogether. They serve to recall conditions which existed in bygone ages, and, while they have a long and significant phylogenetic history, they have lost among living vertebrates all physiological importance.

After closure of the neuro-enteric canal and obliteration of the post-anal gut the alimentary tube ends, during a short period, both cephalad and caudad in a blind pouch. Very soon, however, the ectoderm becomes invaginated at both extremities and finally perforates into the lumen of the intestine, thus establishing the oral and anal communications with the exterior. The anal ectodermal invagination (proctodæum) (Fig. 21), is smaller than the oral (stomadæum) (Fig. 27), but the intestinal tube forms an extensive pouch in the anal region which descends to meet the ectodermal invagination of the proctodæum. The details of the embryonic processes leading to the final establishment of the adult condition are of great interest on account of the pathological importance of abnormal or arrested development in these parts. Failure of the caudal intestinal pouch to establish a communication with the anal invagination, or failure of development in either anal invagination or intestinal pouch, leads to the condition known as atresia ani or imperforate anus, of which there are several varieties.

Before the anal opening forms the primitive caudal intestine receives from above the stalk of the *allantois*, while the Wolffian duct, the canal of the embryonic excretory apparatus, also opens into it. The renal bud on the Wolffian duct in Fig. 28 indicates the beginning development of the permanent kidney (metanephros), and the proximal portion of the allantoic stalk is destined to form by a spindle-shaped enlargement the future urinary bladder (Fig. 28). The caudal gut has as yet no anal opening. Ventrad of the tail end of the embryo the ectoderm presents at this time a depression (Fig. 21). The ectoderm lining the bottom of this anal fossa or depression is separated by a little mesoderm tissue from the entodermal lining of the blind pouch of the caudal gut. Ectoderm and entoderm in this region with the intervening mesodermal layer form the *cloacal membrane* (Fig. 21).

Development of Cloaca.—The entodermal pouch or prolongation sent down from the end-gut to meet the anal invagination enlarges and dilates to form a short wide piece of the intestinal tube into which open on the one hand the urinary and sexual ducts of the

5

genito-urinary system, while it receives on the other the termination of the *end-gut proper* (Figs. 28 and 29).

FIG. 23.—Genito-urinary tract and cloaca of *Iguana tuberculata*, ♀. (Columbia University Museum, No. 1846.)

This is the permanent condition of the terminal openings of the alimentary and genito-urinary tracts in the lower vertebrates. It is found in certain fishes, in all amphibia, reptiles and birds, and occurs also in one order of mammals, the monotremes. In man and mammals generally the anal orifice is separated from the genito-urinary opening, lying dorsad of the same and provided with special sphincters. Only in the monotremes do the anus and the genito-urinary tract open into a common cloaca surrounded by a sphincter common to the anal and genito-urinary openings (sphincter cloacæ). In birds, reptiles, amphibia and many fishes (especially the Plagiostomata) this cloacal formation is the rule. In many fishes, especially the Teleosts, the anus and the genito-urinary openings are separate, as in mammals, but their position is reversed, the anus being ventral, while the genito-urinary opening is placed dorsally.

Fig. 23 shows the cloaca in a female specimen of *Iguana tuberculata*. The ventral wall of the cloaca has been divided to the left of the median line and turned over to the right, carrying with it the cloacal opening of the bladder. The termination of the alimentary canal opens into the cloaca from above.

A transverse fold of the mucosa separates this upper compartment of the cloaca (*coprodæum*) from a lower space (*urodæum*) which receives in its dorsal wall the openings of the two oviducts and immediately above them—upon two papillæ—the openings of the ureters, while the ventral wall contains the cloacal opening of the bladder.

The right ovary has been removed—to show the abdominal opening of the right oviduct—by dividing the mesovarian peritoneal fold.

FIG. 24.—Genito-urinary tract and cloaca of the hen, *Gallus bankiva*. (Columbia University Museum, No. 1208.)

Fig. 24—taken from a preparation of the hen—shows the typical arrangement of the female genito-urinary tract and cloaca in the birds.

The terminal portion of the alimentary canal, in entering the cloaca, forms an expanded upper cloacal compartment for the accumulation of the excreta, called the *coprodæum*.

It is separated by a prominent mucous fold from the central compartment, or *urodæum* which receives the terminations of the two ureters and of the single (left) oviduct. A second fold forms the distal limit of the urodæum and separates it from the lowest cloacal compartment, the *proctodæum*.

FIG. 25.—Genito-urinary tract and cloaca of *Platypus anatinus*, duck-billed platypus. (Columbia University Museum, No. 1802.)

FIG. 26.—Neuro-enteric canal in section of human embryo of 2 mm. (After Spee.)

FIG. 27.—Median section through head of embryo rabbit of 6 mm. (Mihulkovics.)

FIG. 28.—Reconstruction of caudal end of human embryo of 11.5 mm. (four and a half weeks), showing pelvic structures. × 40. (After Keibel.)

FIG. 29.—Reconstruction of caudal end of human embryo of 14 mm. (five weeks). × 20 (After Keibel.)

FIG. 30.—Human female fœtus, 3.4 cm. long, vertex-coccygeal measure. The external perineal folds separate the anal invagination from the uro-genital opening. (Kollmann.)

Fig. 25 shows the male genito-urinary tract and the cloaca in the monotreme, *Platypus anatinus*. The cloaca is a spacious sac formed by the confluence of the rectum and the genito-urinary sinus.

The penis, consisting of two large cavernous bodies, is contained in a fibrous sac which arises from the junction of the genito-urinary sinus and the cloaca, and is continued into the ventral wall of the cloaca near its termination by an opening through which the penis can pass into the cloaca and beyond the external cloacal aperture.

The semen enters the penis at its root through a narrow opening situated close to the junction of genito-urinary sinus and cloaca.

For a short period, therefore, the human embryo and the embryos of the higher mammalia present conditions which correspond to the permanent structure of the parts in these lower vertebrates. In human embryos of 11.5 mm. cervico-coccygeal measure (32-33 days) (Fig. 28), the cloaca appears as a short sac continuous dorsad with the intestine, ventrad with the rudiment of the urinary bladder. The larger portion of the caudal gut (postanal gut) has disappeared, having been reduced to a thin epithelial strand which gradually becomes entirely absorbed. Only the proximal portion of the end-gut is used for the development of the cloaca, which, however, at first has no external opening (Fig. 28).

The tail end of the embryo becomes more extended and between it and the umbilical cord an interval appears in which the genital protuberance develops. Behind this point the ventral cloacal wall is formed by the cloacal membrane.

A considerable interval also develops between the points of entrance into the cloaca of the intestine proper and of the allantoic stalk (urinary bladder). The growth of the mesoderm pushes the intestine against the sacral vertebræ, while the stalk of the allantois with the rudimentary urinary bladder is forced against the ventral abdominal wall. These changes prepare the way for the first appearance of the *genito-urinary sinus*. The neck of the embryonic bladder elongates and receives the ducts of the urinary and genital glands (Fig. 29). In embryos of 14 mm. cervico-coccygeal measure (36-37 days) (Figs. 29 and 30), the genito-urinary sinus perforates the cloacal membrane on the ventral aspect of the genital protuberance, forming the *uro-genital cleft*. The rectum remains closed for a few days longer. The perforation is preceded by the formation of a transverse ectodermal reduplication, producing a depression called the *transverse anal fissure*. This depression increases in depth until a distinct anal invagination results, known as the *proctodæum*, which grows as a funnel-shaped fossa toward the blind termination of the endgut. In embryos of 25 mm. cervico-coccygeal measure (8½-9 weeks) the intestine still ends in a blind pouch. The anus is, therefore, independent of the end-gut in its development. It is derived from the ectoderm and its production is analogous to the formation of the oral cavity by means of the ectodermal invagination called the *stomadæum*.

Finally the cloaca is converted into a ventral tube from which part of the urinary bladder, the urethra and genito-urinary sinus develop, and a dorsal tube from which the *rectum* is derived. This double disposition of the cloaca is accomplished by gradual changes in the entoderm and mesoderm. The entoderm proliferates until a partition is formed which separates the two divisions of the cloacal tube from each other, and the mesoderm likewise increases, surrounding the newly formed entodermal tubes with tissue from which the muscles, connective tissue and blood vessels of the parts are derived (Figs. 28 and 29).

This partition, the *septum uro-rectale*, develops symmetrically on each side, appearing first as paired folds on the right and left sides called the *internal perineal folds* (Figs. 28 and 29). When these folds have reached the cloacal membrane they complete the separation of the cloaca into two adjacent canals. Each of these canals is still closed caudad by its respective portion of the cloacal membrane, now divided into an *anal* and *uro-genital* segment. These two portions of the original cloacal membrane become perforated separately, the uro-genital before the anal. Hence the external opening of the uro-genital sinus is the first to appear, to be followed by the anal perforation. The internal perineal folds are supplemented by the formation of similar external folds, ridges of mesoderm tissue which surround the anal orifice in the form of a low wall and thus deepen the anal ectodermal invagination into the fossa of the proctodæum.

FIG. 31.—Section of pelvis of human fœtus, showing atresia recti. (Esmarch.)

These developmental stages in the formation of the end-gut are of importance because they offer the explanation of the pathological conditions which result from an arrest of development and from the failure of either the uro-genital or anal opening to form in the usual manner. These malformations must date back to an early stage, and probably have their inception in disturbances occurring in the normal development between the 15th and 23d day (embryos of 3-6 mm.). Perhaps in some cases of atresia there may be a secondary obliteration of a previously formed opening. In Fig. 31 the proctodæum persists but the perforation of the anal membrane into the end-gut has not occurred. The ectoderm of the anal fossa and the intestinal entoderm remain separated by a transverse mesodermal partition. Different degrees of this malformation are observed. The layer separating the skin from the blind end of the rectum may be so thin that the meconium contained in the latter can be felt through it. On the other hand the rectum may terminate high up in a blind pouch, which is separated from the skin by a distance of several centimeters.

We may now briefly consider the genetic, histological and mechanical conditions which the above-outlined course of development imposes on the alimentary tract.

The ectoderm forms the superficial covering of the embryo and in the dorsal axial line develops the medullary groove which subsequently becomes converted into the cerebro-spinal axis by closure of the medullary plates and inclusion of the neural tube within the surrounding mesoblast (Fig. 18). The entoderm forms the epithelial lining of the interior of the alimentary canal and its appendages and derivatives (Fig. 19). The mesoderm furnishes the skeletal, muscular and vascular systems. At first single, like the two remaining layers of the blastoderm, the mesoderm splits early on each side of the chorda dorsalis into two layers, including between them spaces which after coalescence form the *primitive pleuro-peritoneal* or *body-cavity* (Fig. 20). One of these mesodermal layers bounding this space becomes closely connected with the ectoderm, forming the *somatopleure* or body wall, while the other joins the entoderm to complete the wall of the alimentary canal, forming the *splanchnopleure*. In the course of further development the edges of these two layers approach each other ventrally in the median line and finally fuse.

The products of this fusion are two epithelial tubes, one included within the other, with walls reinforced by tissue derived from the two layers of the mesoderm. The internal or entodermal tube is of much smaller diameter than the outer or ectodermal tube, but much longer. The walls of the two tubes are placed in contact with each other by their mesodermal elements dorsally in the axial line, but elsewhere are separated from each other by the body-cavity (except in the region of the ventral mesogastrium).

The splanchnopleure is not so wide as the somatopleure. As it closes in the ventral median line it includes the deepest or entodermal layer. It now forms a tube whose walls are composed superficially of mesoderm (splanchnopleure) while the lumen is lined by epithelium derived from the entoderm. This tube is the *primitive enteric* or *alimentary canal*. The somatopleuric layers bounding the body cavity take a wider sweep and after they have united ventrally in the median line they embrace a much more extensive space, the *primitive body cavity* or *cœlom*. The walls of this space are largely made up of the skeletal and muscular elements developed from the mesoderm of the somatopleure, covered superficially by the common ectodermal investment of the body. It will be seen that the enteric tube thus becomes included within the wider and more capacious cœlom cavity.

Both the somatic and the splanchnic leaf of the mesoderm consist at first solely of a layer of flattened epithelial cells, the mesothelium. But very early this tissue is increased to form a massive layer by direct development from the mesothelium. The new mesodermal cells thus produced constitute the *mesenchyma*, which includes the whole of the mesoderm of the embryo except the mesothelial lining of the cœlom. The cells of the mesenchyma, connected with each other and with the mesothelial cells by protoplasmic processes, are not as close together as in an epithelium and do not form a continuous membrane. By migration and multiplication a large mass of mesodermal tissue is produced which fills the entire space between the mesothelium and the primary germ layers. The mesenchymal tissue between the mesothelium and the ectoderm forms the mass of the skeletal, muscular and vascular systems. The mesenchymal tissue between the mesothelium and the entoderm forms an important constituent of the alimentary canal and of its appendages. The entoderm furnishes the internal epithelial lining of the tube upon which the performance of the specific physiological function of the entire apparatus depends. This epithelial tube is covered from without by the splanchnic mesoderm. The mesodermal elements thus added to the enteric entodermal tube consist of connective tissue and muscular fibers. The latter, arranged in the

8

form of circular and longitudinal layers, control the contractility of the tube and regulate the propulsion of the contents. The connective tissue of the splanchnic mesoderm appears as an intermediate layer uniting the epithelial lining and the muscular walls. Situated thus between the mucous and muscular coats of the intestine this layer is known as the *submucosa*. It contains, imbedded in its tissue, the glandular elements of the intestine derived from the entodermal epithelium, and the blood vessels, lymphatics and nerves. The second chief function of the splanchnic and somatic mesoderm is the production of the serous membrane investing the body cavity and its contents from the mesothelium lining the primitive cœlom. This mesothelial tissue, differentiated as a layer of flattened cells, lines the interior of the body cavity and covers the superficial aspect of the enteric tube. By subsequent partition of the common cœlom the great serous membranes of the adult, the pleuræ, pericardium and peritoneum, are developed from it.

FIG. 32.—Schematic diagrams, illustrating the vertebral mesentery. *A*.earlier; *B*. later condition. (Minot.)

The entodermal enteric tube is, as already stated, closely attached at an early period along its dorsal surface to the axial rod of mesoderm containing the chorda dorsalis immediately ventrad of the neural canal. In the earliest stages, just after the splanchnopleure and somatopleure have closed to complete the alimentary tube and body cavity, the remnant of these layers extends between the ventral abdominal wall and the ventral surface of the intestine forming a partition which divides the body into a right and left half. (Fig. 32, *A*.) For the most part this primitive connection between the ventral abdominal wall and the intestinal tube is lost very early. The stomach, however, is always connected by a ventral mesogastrium, from which the lesser omentum is derived, to the ventral body wall. The disappearance of the ventral mesentery caudad of this point establishes the condition indicated in Fig. 32, *B*. The entodermal tube and the surrounding splanchnic mesoderm forming the intestinal canal is attached along its dorsal surface to the axial mesoderm of the dorsal mid-line. The primitive mesothelial peritoneum is reflected along this line from the internal surface of the body wall upon the ventral and lateral surfaces of the intestine. The cœlom of one side communicates ventrad of the intestine with the cœlom of the opposite side. Hence by the disappearance of the ventral mesentery caudad of the stomach the paired body-cavities have become fused into a single abdominal cavity—while cephalad the original division into right and left halves is maintained by the portion of the ventral mesentery which attaches the stomach to the ventral abdominal wall. The mesodermal tissue which at this time attaches thealimentary tube along its entire extent to the dorsal wall of the cœlom carries the primitive embryonic arterial vessel, the aorta. This vessel supplies a series of small branches to the intestine, which reach the same by passing ventrad imbedded in the mesoderm connecting the tube to the dorsal body wall.

With the further development of the alimentary canal a gradual elongation of this connecting band of mesoderm and of the contained vessels is observed, the tube itself gradually receding from the vertebral axis. The early broad attachment is replaced by a narrower stalk into which the mesoderm is drawn out. With this narrowing in the transverse and elongation in the sagittal direction the connecting tissue assumes the character of a thin membrane with two free serous surfaces, including the intestinal vessels imbedded between them. Coincident with this elongation of the enteric attachment and its narrowing in the transverse direction the primitive intestine becomes more completely invested by the serous lining membrane of the cœlom cavity. In this stage we can speak of the double-layered membrane attaching the tube to the dorsal body wall and carrying the intestinal blood-vessels as the primitive dorsal mesentery. The intestinal canal itself is invested by serous membrane except along a narrow strip of its dorsal border where the mesentery is attached and where the vessels reach the intestine. We can now distinguish the serous lining membrane of the abdominal cavity, derived from the mesothelium of the splanchnic and somatic mesoderm as the *peritoneum*. The membrane presents the following topographical subdivisions:

1. *Parietal Peritoneum*, lining the inner surface of the abdominal walls.
2. *Visceral Peritoneum*, investing the external surface of the intestine and its derivatives.

9

3. *Mesenteric Peritoneum*, connecting these two, carrying the intestinal blood vessels and lymphatics and acting as a suspensory support to the alimentary canal.

The dorsal mesentery in fishes, amphibia and reptiles contains smooth muscular fibers derived from the mesoderm. These bands of smooth muscle fibers are also encountered, though less well developed, in the mesentery of birds and mammals. The so-called "suspensory muscle of the duodenum" belongs to this category. It consists of a few strands of unstriped muscular and fibrous tissue which passes from the præaortal tissue around the origin of the superior mesenteric artery and cœliac axis to the duodeno-jejunal angle. Fasciculi from this band may penetrate into the root of the mesentery (Gegenbaur).

Similar muscular fasciculi have been observed in the peritoneal folds of the ileo-cæcal junction (Luschka) and in the mesorectum—forming in the latter situation the recto-coccygeal muscles of Treitz, and in the female the recto-uterine muscles.

In its earlier stages the primitive common mesentery forms a membrane which carries the intestinal blood vessels between its two layers, surrounds the embryonic alimentary canal and attaches the same to the ventral aspect of the chorda dorsalis and aorta. This is the permanent condition in many of the lower vertebrates in which the intestinal tube is suspended by a simple dorsal mesentery, a condition which is repeated by the embryos of man and the higher vertebrates. From this primitive common mesentery are derived, by further development, displacement and adhesion, all the other mesenteries, omenta and peritoneal folds of the adult. The character and degree of these subsequent changes is determined by the increase in length and change in position of the intestine and the growth of large organs, like liver, spleen and pancreas. Many portions of the intestinal canal, at first suspended by the mesentery and freely movable within the abdominal cavity, become later, by secondary adhesion, firmly connected with adjacent portions of the tube or with the abdominal parietes.

In certain of the lower vertebrates (fishes) large sections of the intestine lie entirely free within the abdomen, their only connection with the parietes being afforded by the blood vessels. This condition depends upon *absorption* of the original mesentery. A similar process, though much more circumscribed, is observed in the omenta of many mammals, which appear perforated at several points.

FIG. 33.—Schema of alimentary canal and accessory organs, derived from same. (After Bonnet.)

FIG. 34.—Reconstruction of alimentary canal of human embryo of 4.2 mm. × 24. (After His.)

Derivatives of the Entodermal Intestinal Tube.—The entodermal epithelium is physiologically the characteristic element of the alimentary canal. Besides lining the entire internal surface of the tube it gives rise by budding and protrusion from the intestinal canal to a series of organs which from the mode of their development must be regarded as diverticular or derivatives of the alimentary canal (Figs. 33, 34, and 35). These organs, proceeding in order cephalo-caudad, are the following:

The   salivary   glands.
Thymus   and   thyroid.
The   lungs.
Pancreas.
Liver.

The epithelium of all these structures is derived from the primitive entoderm of the intestinal tube, except the epithelium of the salivary glands, which, being derived from the stomadæal invagination, is ectodermal in character. We have previously noted the general history and appearance of the yolk-sac and its connection by means of the vitello-intestinal duct with the intestine. In contradistinction to the adult organs just noted the yolk-sac or umbilical vesicle is merely a temporary embryonal appendage to the alimentary canal. It also differs from them in the fact that it is not an extension or budding from the completed intestinal tube, like the liver and pancreas, but indicates, by the implantation of the duct (Fig. 21), the last point at which closure of the intestinal canal takes place, when after obliteration of the duct the separation of the intestine from the yolk-sac is completed.

10

The segment of the primitive alimentary canal cephalad of the attachment of the vitello-intestinal duct gives rise to the pharynx, œsophagus, stomach, proximal portion of small intestine proper and its derivatives, the liver and pancreas.

FIG. 35.—Reconstruction of alimentary canal of human embryo of 7 mm. (twenty-eight days). × 12. (After His.)

FIG. 36.—Reconstruction of alimentary canal of human embryo of thirty-five days (13.8 mm.). × 8. (After His.)

The portion situated caudad of the duct produces the rest of the small and all of the large intestine (Figs. 33 and 35). At times in man and other mammals (cat) the vitello-intestinal duct does not become absorbed, but persists and continues to develop as a part of the small intestine, forming the blind pouch or appendage known as *Meckel's diverticulum* (Figs. 37 and 38). This diverticulum may vary in length from 1.5 to 15 cm. It either projects freely into the abdominal cavity as a pouch arising from the convex border of the small intestine opposite to the mesenteric attachment, or else it reaches the abdominal wall at the umbilicus and is attached to the same. In a few instances it has not terminated in a blind pouch, but has remained open at the umbilicus, in which case the aperture discharges intestinal contents. Sometimes the process of obliteration which normally leads to the absorption of the vitello-intestinal duct extends to the adjoining segment of the small intestine, resulting in obliteration of the intestinal lumen and consequent obstruction at this point.

FIG. 37.—Human adult ileum with Meckel's diverticulum. Ileo-diverticular serous fold and persistent omphalo-mesenteric artery. (Columbia University Museum, No. 1803.)

FIG. 38.—Human adult ileum, with Meckel's diverticulum. (Columbia University Museum, No. 745.)

The intestinal opening of the diverticulum is situated at a varying distance above the ileo-colic junction, ranging from 27.5 cm. to 290 cm., with an average of 107 cm.

While the obliteration and complete absorption of the duct is normal in nearly all vertebrates, a remnant persists in some birds, in which a short cæcal pouch (*diverticulum cæcum vitelli*) is found at about the middle of the small intestine. A portion of the vitello-intestinal duct thus persists throughout life in some wading and swimming birds. Figs. 39 and 40 show this condition in the small intestine of *Urinator lumme* and *imber*, the red-throated loon and the great northern diver. In other birds, however, such as birds of prey, song birds, etc., the duct is absorbed and disappears completely.

FIG. 39.—Small intestine of the red-throated loon, *Urinator lumme*, showing persistent cæcal pouch, the remnant of the vitelline duct. (Columbia University Museum, No. 997.)

FIG. 40.—Small intestine of great northern diver, *Urinator imber*, with cæcal pouch, the remnant of the vitelline duct. (Columbia University Museum, No. 77, 1578.)

In order to complete the embryological history of the alimentary canal it is necessary to take brief account of another structure derived from it, namely the *allantois*. Its significance to the adult organism is seen in connection with the genito-urinary tract, the urinary bladder being formed by its persistent portion. In the embryo, however, it has important nutritive and respiratory functions. In the embryos of the higher vertebrates nutrition depends only in the earliest stages upon the yolk-sac of the ovum, over which a vascular network extends.

FIG. 41.—Diagram illustrating the later stages in the formation of the mammalian fœtal membranes. (Heisler, modified from Roule.)

Very soon the caudal portion of the primitive intestine develops a vascular sac-like outgrowth (Figs. 21 and 41). This pouch forms the *allantois*. It is intimately connected with embryonal respiration, and probably also forms a reservoir which receives the secretion of the primitive kidney. This foreshadows the final destiny of the proximal intra-abdominal

11

portion of the allantoic sac which persists and is converted into the urinary bladder of the adult.

The allantois is present in Amphibia but is very small. In Amniota[1] it is large and grows around the embryo. In those of the higher vertebrates which are developed within an egg (reptiles, birds and monotremes) the sac of the allantois comes to lie beneath the egg-shell and acts as a respiratory organ. In the higher mammalia, developed within the uterus, the allantois becomes attached by vascular villi to the uterine wall and establishes a vascular connection between the fœtal and maternal blood vessels. In this way the *allantoic placenta* is formed (Fig. 41). The placenta, as just stated, is absent in the monotremes and is only slightly developed in marsupials, in which animals the fœtus develops to maturity in the marsupial pouch after leaving the uterus. These animals are therefore distinguished as *Aplacentalia* from the remaining higher mammals in which the allantoic placenta develops and which are hence called the *Placentalia*.

Summary.—To recapitulate, therefore, the intestinal tube gives origin to two kinds of appendages or derivatives:

1. Organs of the adult body, derived by budding from the alimentary entodermal epithelium, in the form of pouch-like diverticula which follow the glandular type of development and become secondarily associated with mesodermal elements. These organs are again of two kinds:

(*a*) *Organs which retain their original connection with the lumen of the digestive canal:*

The salivary glands,

The liver,   Connected by their ducts with the digestive canal.
The pancreas,
The lungs,

which open by means of the trachea and the laryngeal aperture into the pharyngeal cavum.

(*b*) *Organs which lose their primitive connection with the alimentary canal.*

Thymus and Thyroid Gland.

2. Embryonic appendages of the alimentary tract.

(*a*) The vitello-intestinal or omphalo-mesenteric duct and the yolk-sac or umbilical vesicle. This structure does not form as an extension from the intestinal tube after the same has been closed by coalescence of the splanchnopleure in the ventral mid-line, but is the result of the folding in of the layers of the embryonic germinal area, by means of which the body-rudiment is constricted off from the yolk-sac. The reduced channel of communication forms the vitello-intestinal duct. In the vast majority of vertebrates this disappears completely by absorption in the course of further development. It may persist in part abnormally as Meckel's diverticulum. In a few birds its proximal portion remains normally as a small blind pouch attached to the free border of the small intestine.

FIG. 42.—Genito-urinary tract and cloaca of *Iguana tuberculata*, ♀. (Columbia University Museum, No. 1846.)

(*b*) The allantois. This is a hollow outgrowth from the embryonic intestinal canal of the higher vertebrates, performing important functions in connection with the early nutrition of the embryo. In the course of subsequent development its proximal portion, situated within the abdominal cavity, becomes converted into the urinary bladder. In mammals it loses its original connection with the intestinal canal and is assigned entirely to the genito-urinary tract. In some of the lower vertebrates, amphibia and reptiles it retains its connection with the ventral wall of the cloaca throughout life. (See Fig. 42, genito-urinary tract of *Iguana tuberculata*.)

After the intestinal canal has become separated from the yolk-sac it forms at first a straight tube, running cephalo-caudad beneath the chorda dorsalis. In most forms, however, the intestine grows much more rapidly in length than the body-cavity of the embryo in which it is contained. Hence the intestine is forced to form coils or convolutions.

The entire alimentary canal, from the mouth to the anus, can be separated into the following divisions and subdivisions:

12

I. Foregut, including

1.	The	oral	cavity.
2.		The	pharynx.
3.		The	œsophagus.

4. The stomach.

II. Midgut, closely associated at its beginning with the liver and pancreas.

It extends between the pyloric extremity of the stomach and the beginning of the last segment, the endgut, frequently separated from both by ring-like aggregations of the circular muscular fibers and corresponding projections of the mucous membrane (pyloric and ileo-colic valves).

The midgut is usually the longest portion of the intestinal tube.

III. Endgut, the last segment of the intestinal canal, courses through the pelvic portion of the body cavity. From this short end-piece are developed: (1) The colon, sigmoid flexure and rectum; (2) the cloaca with the uro-genital sinus and the duct of the allantois.

PART I.
ANATOMY OF THE PERITONEUM AND ABDOMINAL CAVITY.

For the purpose of studying the adult human peritoneum it is in the first place absolutely necessary to obtain a correct appreciation of the disposition of the chief viscera within the abdominal cavity and of their mutual relations. In the second place the visceral vascular supply of the abdomen must be carefully considered in order to correctly appreciate certain important relations of the peritoneal membrane.

A review of the visceral contents of the abdomen shows that we have to deal chiefly with the divisions of the alimentary tract below the œsophagus and the structures directly derived from the same, as liver and pancreas, or associated topographically with the alimentary canal, as the spleen. Portions of the urinary and reproductive systems situated within the abdominal and pelvic cavities will also require consideration.

The digestive apparatus as a whole presents, in the first place, a segment designed to convey the food to the stomach, the œsophagus—supplemented in mammalia by the special apparatus of the mouth and pharynx, in which the food is mechanically prepared for digestion by chewing and mixed with the secretion of the salivary glands.

The *digestive apparatus proper*, succeeding to the œsophagus, is usually divisible into two sections differing in function and structure.

1. The STOMACH, a short sac-like dilatation, in which chiefly nitrogenous material is digested.

2. The SMALL INTESTINE, a long and usually much convoluted narrow tube, chiefly devoted to the digestion of starches, fats and sugars, and to the absorption of the digested matters.

In some of the lower vertebrates, as the *Cyclostomata* (Fig. 43), *Esox*, *Belone*, etc., among fishes (Fig. 48), *Necturus* and *Proteus* among amphibians (Figs. 50 and 51), the separation of the digestive portion of the alimentary tract into stomach and small intestine is not clearly defined (vide infra, p. 43).

FIG. 43.—Entire alimentary canal of the lamprey, *Petromyzon marinus*, below the pericardium. (Columbia University Museum, No. 1575.)

FIG. 44.—Schematic diagram representing three stages in the differentiation of the mammalian digestive tract: A. Early undifferentiated stage, in which the entire canal appears as a tube of uniform calibre. B. Spindle-shaped gastric dilatation. C. Typical mammalian gastric dilatation.

FIG. 45.—Reconstruction of human embryo. 1, 2, 3, 4, Gill-pouches. (After Fol.)

A distinct digestive segment may even be entirely wanting, owing to its failure to differentiate from the œsophagus on the one hand and from the endgut on the other. In such forms the entire digestive canal appears as a tube of uniform caliber extending from mouth to anus. It is necessary to begin with these simple structural conditions in order to obtain a clear conception of the disposition of the viscera in the adult human abdomen.

13

Such simple arrangement of the alimentary tract is found in the embryo of man and of the higher vertebrates, and similar rudimentary types are encountered, as the permanent condition, in some of the lower forms. These latter are especially valuable for purposes of study, because they afford an opportunity of examining directly, as macroscopic objects, structural conditions which are found only as temporary embryonal stages during the development of the higher mammalia (Fig. 43).

In the early stages the alimentary tract of the mammalian embryo consists of a straight tube of nearly uniform caliber (Fig. 44, *A*), extending from the pharynx to the cloaca, along the median line in the dorsal region of the body cavity, connected with the ventral aspect of the axial mesoderm by a membranous fold forming the primitive common dorsal mesentery. Subsequently differentiation of this simple tube into successive segments takes place, marked by differences in shape and caliber and in histological structure.

The first indication of the future stomach appears early, in human embryos of from 5-6 days (Figs. 44, *B*, and 45; for later embryonal stomach forms compare also Figs. 33, 35 and 36), as a small spindle-shaped dilatation of a portion of the primitive entodermal tube, placed in the median plane, dorsad of the embryonic outgrowth of the liver, between it and the œsophagus. The appearance of this dilatation marks the separation of the proximal cephalic part (pharynx and œsophagus) from the distal caudal (intestinal) portion of the primitive alimentary canal.

Further growth of the stomach takes place chiefly along the dorsal margin of the dilatation, rendering the same more convex. The ventral border develops to a less degree and in the course of further and more complete differentiation the dorsal margin of the future stomach assumes even at this period the character of the greater curvature, while the opposite ventral margin, the future lesser curvature, following the dilatation of the tube dorsad, becomes in turn concave (Fig. 44, *C*).

FIG. 46.—Alimentary canal of human embryo of 5 mm. × 15. (Reconstruction after His.)

The early spindle-shaped dilatation has therefore assumed the general shape of the adult organ. This differentiation of greater and lesser curvature begins to appear in embryos of 5 mm. (Fig. 46) and is very well marked in embryos of 12.5 mm.,Fig. 36, of an embryo of five weeks, indicates the adult form of the stomach clearly.

It will, however, be noted that the œsophageal entrance is still at the cephalic extremity of the rudimentary stomach, while the pyloric transition to the intestine occupies the distal caudal point, under cover of the liver, and turns with a slight bend dorsad and to the right to pass into the duodenum. The future greater curvature is directed dorsad and a little to the left toward the vertebral column, while the concave lesser curvature is turned ventrad and a little to the right toward the ventral abdominal wall. At this time there is but little indication of the subsequent extension of the organ to the left of the œsophageal entrance to form the great cul-de-sac or fundus of the adult stomach.

In this stage of its development the stomach therefore presents ventral and dorsal borders, and right and left surfaces, while the continuity of its lumen with the adjacent segments of the alimentary canal appears as a proximal or cephalic œsophageal and a distal or caudal intestinal opening.

COMPARATIVE ANATOMY OF FOREGUT AND STOMACH.

A serial review of this portion of the alimentary tract in vertebrates forms one of the most interesting and instructive chapters in comparative anatomy.

FIG. 47.—*Gallus canis*, dog-shark, ♂. Genito-urinary tract and cloaca *in situ*. The foregut has been divided just caudad of the communication with the oral cavity. (Columbia University Museum, No. 1694.)

Not only is every embryonal stage in the development of the higher mammalia represented permanently in the adult structure of some of the lower types, but the far-reaching influence of function and of the physiological demands on the structure of this portion of the digestive tract is strikingly illustrated by the numerous and marked modifications which are encountered.

The foregut, strictly speaking, is in mammals separated from the oral cavity by the musculo-membranous fold of the soft palate and uvula. In all other vertebrates except the crocodile, the oral cavity and foregut pass into each other without sharp demarcation (Fig. 47). In some of the lower vertebrates the alimentary canal never advances beyond the condition of a simple straight tube of nearly uniform caliber. There is no gastric dilatation and hence no differentiation of a stomach properly speaking. Such for example is the case in some teleost fishes, as the pickerel (Fig. 48). In these forms we have to deal with the persistence of the early embryonic pregastric stage of the higher types, before the simple alimentary tube is differentiated by the appearance of the distinct gastric dilatation.

In the *Cyclostomata* (Fig. 43) the intestinal canal passes through the body in a perfectly straight line and the three segments (mid-, fore- and hindgut) are not clearly differentiated.

In the *Ammocœtes* the foregut begins behind the wide branchial basket, dorsad of the heart, with a narrow entrance, which is succeeded by a dilated segment. The entrance of the hepatic duct separates fore- and midgut.

In *Amphioxus* the branchial pouch passes with a slight constriction directly into the gut which extends through the body-cavity in a straight line.

The narrow segment is usually regarded as the "œsophagus." This is followed by a slightly dilated segment, the "stomach," into which a blind pouch enters. This cæcal pouch is usually considered as a *hepatic* diverticulum (Fig. 49).

But even in these rudimentary forms the point where the liver develops from the entodermal intestinal tube marks the separation of fore- and midgut. The stomach, when it develops, is situated cephalad of the entrance of the hepatic duct into the intestine. The section cephalad of the duct opening may be very short, and the food digested further on in the intestinal tube. Consequently a function which in these lower vertebrates is assigned to the midgut becomes transferred in the higher forms to a specialized segment of the foregut, situated cephalad of the hepato-enteric duct. This segment is the . . .

FIG. 48.—Alimentary canal of *Belone*, pickerel. (Nuhn.)	FIG. 49.—*Amphioxus*, dissected from the ventral side. The relatively enormous pharynx occupies more than half the length of the body. The walls are separated by the gill-clefts, and the parallel gill-bars abut at the midventral line on the *endostyle*. (Willey, after Rathke.)	FIG. 50.—*Necturus maculatus*, mud-puppy. Alimentary canal and appendages. (Columbia University Museum, No. 1454.)	FIG. 51.—Alimentary canal of *Proteus anguineus*. (Nuhn.)

STOMACH.

The distribution of the vagus nerve finds its explanation in this derivation of the stomach. The primitive foregut is formed by the passage between the branchial cavity and the midgut, and is within the area supplied by the vagus. Hence when the stomach develops from the foregut, as a specialized segment of the same, it is supplied by vagus branches. The vertebrate stomach varies greatly in size and shape.

The type-form is presented by a longitudinal spindle-shaped dilatation of the foregut, which retains its fœtal vertical position in the long axis of the body. An example of this form, which is encountered among fishes and amphibia, is presented by the alimentary tube of *Proteus anguineus* and *Necturus maculatus* (Figs. 50 and 51). Since this condition is common to all vertebrates in the earliest fœtal period it can be designated as the fœtal or primitive stomach form. All others appear as secondary derivatives from this typical early condition.

The influences which bring about such derivations and modifications may be enumerated as follows:

1. The habitual amount of food required by the animal.

2. The volume and digestible character of the food.

FIG. 52.—Alimentary canal of *Coluber natrix*. (Nuhn.)

3. The size and shape of the abdominal cavity in which the stomach is contained.

4. Structural modifications designed to increase the action of the gastric juice on the food contained in the stomach.

15

5. The assumption, on part of the stomach, of functions which are usually relegated to other organs.

Most of the individual stomach forms encountered among vertebrates owe their production to several of these influences acting in conjunction.

We may group the main types as follows:

1. Stomach Forms Depending on the Influence exerted by the Habitual Amount of Food required by the Animal.—The greater the activity of tissue changes is, the greater will be the amount of food required and the more pronounced will be the gastric dilatation of the alimentary canal. Hence in the higher vertebrates generally the stomach appears as a large and more sac-like dilatation than in lower forms, such as fishes and amphibia and some reptilia, in which the stomach is usually smaller and fœtal in shape, forming a slight longitudinal dilatation situated in the long axis of the body. An example is seen in the stomach of *Coluber natrix* (Fig. 52). Frequently this slight dilatation is scarcely differentiated from the œsophagus at the cephalic and from the small intestine at the caudal end. Many batrachians and perennibranchiates possess this form among the amphibia. It is also encountered in the pickerels, the *Cyprini*, and in *Labrus* among fishes, and in some saurians and ophidia among reptiles. It constitutes a slight advance in development over the earliest stage represented, as we have seen, by the nearly uniform and undifferentiated alimentary tube of amphioxus and the cyclostomata.

FIG. 53.—Human adult. Mucous surface of œsophageo-gastric junction. (Columbia University Museum, No. 1842.)

FIG. 54.—Human adult. Pyloro-duodenal junction and pyloric valve in section. (Columbia University Museum, No. 1842.)

FIG. 55.—Series of sections showing human pyloric valve and gastro-duodenal junction:

1. Stomach of fœtus at term in section.
2. Adult pyloric valve, gastric surface.
3. Adult pyloric valve and gastro-duodenal junction in section.
4. Fœtal gastro-duodenal junction in section. Entrance of biliary and pancreatic ducts on summit of papilla of duodenum. (Columbia University Museum, No. 1851.)

This transition of the fœtal form to the more advanced secondary types of the stomach is marked by the development of two important structural features:

(*a*) The separation in the interior of the canal of the stomach from the intestine by the appearance of a ring-shaped valve, the *pyloric valve*. This is produced by an aggregation of the circular muscular fibers of the intestine at this point, and causes a projection of the mucous membrane into the lumen of the canal. It begins to appear in the fishes (pickerel, sturgeon, etc.), is found in most amphibia and is regularly present in the stomach of the higher vertebrates. (Figs. 54 and 55.) A good example of the ring-shaped plate of the pylorus with central circular opening produced by the aggregation of the circular muscular fibers is afforded by the view of the interior of the cormorant's stomach given in Fig. 69. The opposite or œsophageal extremity of the stomach is less well differentiated from the afferent tube of the œsophagus.

There is no aggregation of muscular circular fibers in this situation and no valve. Superficially the external longitudinal muscular fibers of the œsophagus pass continuously and without demarcation into the superficial gastric muscular layer. The separation between œsophagus and stomach is, however, marked on the mucous surface by a well-defined line along which the flat, smooth and glistening œsophageal tesselated epithelium passes into the granular cuboidal epithelium of the gastric mucous membrane. The œsophageo-gastric junction in the adult human subject is shown in Fig. 53.

(*b*) The pyloric end of the stomach makes an angular bend, while the rest of the organ remains in the original vertical position in the long axis of the body. An example of this condition is presented by the stomach of *Scincus ocellatus* (Fig. 56; cf. also Fig. 202).

The purpose of both of these provisions is to retain the gastric contents for a longer time within the stomach. Hence this form is encountered especially in those fishes and amphibians in which the nutritive demands require a more complete digestion of the food taken. This is the case, for example, in *Gobius* (Fig. 57), the plagiostomata (Fig. 58), and many saurians. The same transitory stomach form is even found in some mammals, as the seals. Fig. 59 shows the stomach in *Phoca vitulina*, the harbor seal. With the further increase in the demand for complete digestion of the food the entire stomach assumes a transverse position to the long axis of the body. This may occur while the stomach still retains its primitive tubular form, as in most chelonians (Fig. 60). In others the change in position occurs after the gastric dilatation has assumed the sac-like form, as in many land-turtles, crocodiles, some batrachians and all higher vertebrates (Figs. 61 and 62). This transverse position, at right angles to the long axis of the body, forms the starting point for the derivation of all secondary types of stomach.

FIG. 56.—Alimentary canal of *Scincus ocellatus*. Pyloric extremity of the slightly marked gastric dilatation presents an angular bend. (Nuhn.)

FIG. 57.—Alimentary canal of *Gobius niger*. (Nuhn.)

FIG. 58.—Alimentary canal of shark. (Nuhn.)

FIG. 59.—Stomach of *Phoca vitulina*, harbor seal. (Columbia University Museum, No. 600.)

FIG. 60.—Stomach of *Pseudemys elegans*, pond turtle. (Columbia University Museum, No. 1710.)

FIG. 61.—Stomach of *Chelydra serpentina*, snapping turtle. (Columbia University Museum, No. 1852.)

FIG. 62.—Same in section.

2. Stomach Forms Depending on the Influence Exerted by the Volume and Digestible Character of the Foods.—Vegetable substances usually have a large volume in proportion to the amount of nutritive material which they contain. Meat, on the other hand, contains considerable nutriment in a comparatively small bulk. Hence carnivora (Fig. 63) usually have a smaller stomach than herbivora (Fig. 64).

FIG. 63.—Stomach of *Lutra vulgaris*, otter. (Nuhn.)

FIG. 64.—Stomach of *Equus caballus*, horse. (Nuhn.)

3. Stomach Forms Influenced by Size and Shape of the Abdominal Cavity in which they are Contained.—In animals whose bodies are long and slender, as in snakes (Fig. 52), most saurians (Fig. 56), many tailed batrachians and perennibranchiates (Figs. 50 and 51), many teleosts (Fig. 48), the stomach is likewise usually long and slender in shape, unless special modifying conditions exist. When on the other hand the body is broad and short, as in Lophius (Fig. 65), Pipa (Fig. 66), and most higher vertebrates, the stomach is also broader and more sac-like.

FIG. 65.—Stomach of *Lophius piscatorius*, angler. (Nuhn.)

FIG. 66.—Stomach of *Pipa verrucosa*. (Nuhn.)

4. Stomach Forms Depending on Structural Modifications Designed to Increase the Action of the Gastric Juice on the Food.—This purpose is accomplished:

(*a*) By increasing the source of supply of the gastric juice.

(*b*) By increasing the length of time during which the food remains in the stomach.

FIG. 67.—Stomach of *Castor fiber*, beaver. (Nuhn.)

FIG. 68.—Stomach of *Manatus americanus*, manatee. (Nuhn.)

FIG. 69.—Stomach of *Phalacrocorax dilophus*, double-crested cormorant; section. (Columbia University Museum, No. 67/1804.)

(*a*) The source of supply of the gastric juice is increased by adding to the usual gastric glands of the stomach a special accessory glandular compartment, either placed at the cardia, where the œsophagus enters, as in *Myoxus* or *Castor* (Fig. 67) or attached to the body of the stomach to the left of the cardia, as in the manatee (Fig. 68). The first arrangement is similar to the universal position of the glandular stomach of birds (Fig. 69). In birds, however, the glandular proventriculus is the *only* source of the gastric juice, while in the above-mentioned

17

mammalia (myoxus and beaver) the accessory glandular stomach is merely an addition to the supply derived from the usual gastric glands situated in the body of the organ.

(*b*) The increase of the length of time during which the food remains in the stomach subject to the action of the gastric juice can be accomplished in one of several ways.

1. The stomach, while it retains its general tubular form increases considerably in length and assumes the shape and structure found in the human large intestine. It is partially subdivided by folds projecting into the interior and separating compartments resembling the colic cells of the human large intestine. The time required for the passage of food through the stomach is thus increased and the action of the gastric juice is prolonged and rendered more intense.

Such modifications of the structure of the stomach are encountered in *Semnopithecus* among the monkeys and in the kangaroo, among marsupials (Figs. 70 and 71).

2. The same purpose is accomplished by the development of diverticula from the stomach, in which the food is retained and acted on by the gastric juice for longer periods.

FIG. 70.—Stomach of *Halmaturus derbyanus*, rock kangaroo. (Columbia University Museum, No. 582.)

FIG. 71.—Stomach of *Semnopithecus entellus*, entellus monkey. (Columbia University Museum, No. 62/1805.)

FIG. 72.—Alimentary canal of *Anguilla anguilla*, eel. (Columbia University Museum, No. 1271.)

The herbivora, omnivora and such carnivora as live on animal food difficult of digestion furnish examples of this type of stomach. The same is also found in most teleosts. In the latter the cæcal gastric pouch lies in the long axis of the body, opposite the entrance of the œsophagus. A marked example of this arrangement is seen in the stomach of the eel, *Anguilla anguilla* (Fig. 72).

In other forms, and in the mammalia especially, the blind pouch is developed from the portion of the stomach lying to the left of the œsophageal entrance at the cardia, and is hence placed transversely to the long axis of the body.

This difference in the position of the cul-de-sac is explained by the small transverse measure of the body in teleosts, while the greater amount of available space in the abdominal cavity of mammalia permits of the transverse position of the entire stomach and of the development of the diverticulum from its left extremity.

Most mammals have only a single pouch, whose size varies with the digestibility of the food habitually taken. It is greater in herbivora (Figs. 64 and 73) than in omnivora and carnivora (Figs. 74 and 75). In some of the latter, as *Lutra* (Fig. 63), the cul-de-sac is almost wanting.

FIG. 73.—Stomach of *Lepus cuniculus*, rabbit. (Nuhn.)

FIG. 76.—Stomach of *Erethizon dorsatus*, American porcupine. (Columbia University Museum, No. 358.)

FIG. 74.—Stomach of *Nasua rufa*, coati. (Nuhn.)

FIG. 77.—Stomach of *Cercopithecus cephus*, moustache monkey. (Columbia University Museum, No. 158.)

FIG. 75.—Stomach of *Felis leo*, lion. (Nuhn.)

FIG. 78.—Stomach of *Sus scrofa*, pig. The fundus of the stomach carries a cæcal appendage separated in the interior by a spiral fold of the mucous membrane from the gastric cavity.

In some forms, as the pig, the left extremity of the stomach carries a cæcal appendix with a spiral valve in the interior separating its lumen from the general gastric cavity (Fig. 78). Others have two such cæcal appendices added to the left end of the stomach (Peccary, Fig. 79). These cæcal pouches may arise from the *body* of the stomach, instead of from the left extremity. An example of this condition is furnished by the American manatee (Fig. 68).

18

FIG. 79.—Stomach of *Dicotyles torquatus*, peccary. The fundus is a capacious pouch prolonged ventrally and dorsally into two cæcal appendages resembling the single appendage of the pig's stomach. (Columbia University Museum, No. 1806.)

5. Variations in the Form of the Stomach Depending upon the Assumption by the Stomach of Special Functions, which are Usually Relegated to other Organs.— These functions are the following:

FIG. 80.—*Macacus nemestrinus*, pig-tail macaque monkey; cheek-pouches. (From a fresh dissection.)

FIG. 81.—Stomach of *Cricetus vulgaris*, hamster. (Nuhn.)

(*a*) Storage of food in special receptacles or compartments for subsequent use.

(*b*) Mastication of the food is in some animals accomplished only partly or not at all in the mouth, and is then performed in the stomach. A portion of the stomach is thus converted into an apparatus for mastication.

(*c*) The provisions for these two accessory functions may be combined in the same stomach.

(*a*) Many of the higher vertebrates possess in connection with the alimentary tract additional reservoirs for the storage of food until used. Such reservoirs are found in mammals and birds connected with the oral cavity, as cheek-pouches, or with the œsophagus, such as the crop of the birds (Fig. 88). Fig. 80 shows the development of the cheek-pouches in one of the primates, *Macacus nemestrinus*.

In many mammals reservoirs of similar import are added directly to the stomach and form an integral part of the organ. Examples are furnished by the compound stomachs of many rodents, ruminants, cetaceans and herbivorous edentates. The peculiar appearance of these stomachs is explained if the additional reservoirs are in imagination removed and the digestive stomach proper restored so to speak to the type-form. The proximal or cardiac portion of the stomach in many rodents is devoid of gastric glands and must be interpreted as a storage chamber for food (Fig. 81). The same significance attaches to the corresponding portion of the manatee's stomach (Fig. 68).

Similar contrivances are found in the ruminant stomach. The first and second divisions (rumen and reticulum) are nothing but sac-like gastric reservoirs or pouches, in which the food is collected, to be subsequently returned to the mouth for mastication. When swallowed for the second time the bolus is carried, by the closure of the so-called œsophageal gutter, past the first and second stomach into the digestive apparatus proper (the abomasum) (Figs. 82 and 83). Many ruminants (*e. g.*, *Moschus*) only have these three compartments. Most, however, have four, the leaf stomach or psalterium being intercalated between the retinaculum and the abomasum. The psalterium contains no digestive glands. It may possibly serve for the absorption of the liquid portions of the foods.

FIG. 82.—Stomach of *Ovis aries*, sheep. (Columbia University Museum, No. 1807.)

FIG. 83.—Scheme of ruminant compound stomach. (Nuhn.)

FIG. 84.—Mucous membrane of stomach of *Camelus dromedarius*, dromedary, showing water-cells. (Columbia University Museum, No. 1123.)

FIG. 85.—Stomach of *Phocæna*, porpoise. (Nuhn.)

The rumen or first stomach of the camels and llamas is provided with so-called "water-cells," for the storage of water. These cells are diverticula lined by a continuation of the gastric mucous membrane. The entrance into these compartments can be closed by a sphincter muscle after they are filled with water (Fig. 84).

FIG. 86.—Stomach of *Urinator imber*, red-throated loon. (Columbia University Museum, No. 1808.)

FIG. 87.—Scheme of stomach of granivorous bird. (Nuhn.)

The three stomachs of the cetaceans are similar to those of the ruminants (Fig. 85). The first is a crop-like reservoir for the reception of the food when swallowed. The mucous membrane is entirely devoid of digestive glands. In the dolphins the mucous membrane is provided with a hard horny covering, which serves to break up the food mechanically by trituration. The second stomach and the gut-like pyloric prolongation constituting the third stomach contain gastric glands and are hence digestive in function.

(*b*) Stomach forms, in which a portion of the organ is converted into an apparatus for mastication, are seen especially in birds, in which animals, on account of the absence of teeth, mastication cannot be performed in the mouth.

The stomach of the bird is usually composed of two segments, one placed vertically above the other.

The first appears like an elongated dilatation of the œsophagus, forming the *Proventriculus* or glandular stomach.

The second is larger, round in shape, with very strong and thick muscular walls (Figs. 86 and 87).

The proventriculus furnishes the gastric juice exclusively.

The second or muscular stomach, devoid of gastric glands, functions merely as a masticating apparatus for the mechanical division of the food. The thick muscular walls of this compartment may measure several inches in diameter and carry on the opposed mucous surfaces lining the cavity a hard horny plate with corrugated and roughened surface (Fig. 88). These hard plates are designed to crush the food between them, as between two mill stones. The muscle stomach is best developed in herbivorous birds, while both the muscular wall and the horny plate are much weaker and thinner in carnivore wading and swimming birds (Fig. 89).

FIG. 88.—Œsophagus and stomach of *Gallus bankiva*, hen. (Columbia University Museum, No. 1809.)

FIG. 89.—Stomach of *Botaurus lentiginosus*, bittern. (Columbia University Museum, No. 23/1810.)

FIG. 90.—Stomach of owl sp. (Nuhn.)

FIG. 91.—Stomach of *Ardea cinerea*, heron. (Nuhn.)

FIG. 92.—Stomach of crocodile. (Nuhn.)

In birds of prey, especially in the owls, the stomach walls are scarcely more massive than in other animals, and the mucous membrane is soft and devoid of a horny covering. The glandular and masticatory stomachs are less sharply divided from each other in these forms, and the entire organ conforms more to the general vertebrate type (Fig. 90).

In some birds (herons, storks, etc.) a small rounded third stomach, the so-called pyloric stomach, is placed between the muscle stomach and the pylorus (Fig. 91). It contains no gastric glands, and possibly may function as an additional absorbing chamber.

Among reptiles the stomach of the crocodile resembles the organ in birds (Fig. 92). It is flat and rounded in shape, the muscle wall carries a tendinous plate, and there is a pyloric stomach. There is, however, no glandular stomach or proventriculus, as in birds, and the mucous membrane is not covered by a horny plate, but is soft and contains the peptic glands. Figs. 93 and 94 show the stomach of *Alligator mississippiensis*, in the ventral view and in section.

FIG. 93.—Stomach of *Alligator mississippiensis*. (Columbia University Museum, No. 1811.)

FIG. 94.—Same in section. Thin-walled cardiac segment continues into cavity of pyloric ventriculus.

FIG. 95.—Stomach of *Bradypustridactylus*, three-toed sloth. I. First stomach, devoid of gastric glands, corresponding to rumen of ruminants.

II. Second stomach, the homologue of the ruminant reticulum.

III. Digestive stomach proper, provided with gastric glands connected by a gutter with the œsophagus.

IV. Muscular stomach, the walls formed by a thick muscular plate and provided on the mucous surface with a dense corneous covering for purposes of trituration.

(*c*) The combination of the two accessory functions just described in the same stomach is found in the three-toed sloth (Fig. 95).

There are here two large reservoirs, which correspond to the rumen and retinaculum of the ruminants, and a digestive compartment containing gastric glands, which corresponds to the ruminant abomasum, and is connected by an œsophageal gutter directly with the œsophagus. At the pyloric extremity the muscle wall is greatly increased and the mucous membrane of this portion carries a thick horny covering, forming a masticatory stomach greatly resembling the corresponding structure in the bird. Its function is evidently to complete the mechanical division of the food which has only been partly masticated in the mouth.

The same significance is probably to be attached to the thickened muscular walls which the pyloric segment of the stomach in *Tamandua bivittata*, another edentate, presents (Fig. 96), in strong contrast with the thinner walled cardiac segment and fundus.

FIG. 96.—Stomach of *Tamandua bivittata*, collared ant-eater, (Columbia University Museum, No. 68/1485.)

INTESTINE.

Continuing our consideration of the development of the alimentary canal we find that changes from the simple primitive straight tube below the stomach depend upon two factors:

1. The increase in the length of the intestinal tube, which exceeds relatively the increase in the length of the body cavity in which it is contained.

2. The differentiation into small and large intestine, the development of the cæcum and ileo-cæcal junction, and the development of the accessory digestive glands, liver and pancreas, by budding from the proximal portion of the primitive entodermal intestinal tube.

FIG. 97.—Alimentary canal of human embryo of 5 mm. × 15. (Reconstruction after His.)

FIG. 98.—Schema of human embryonic intestinal canal, with intestinal umbilical loop, but before differentiation of the large and small intestine.

FIG. 99.—Viscera of *Necturus maculatus*, mud-puppy, *in situ*. (Columbia University Museum, No. 1175.)

1. In embryos up to 5 mm. cervico-coccygeal measure (Fig. 97) the intestinal tube follows the body curve without deviation. Subsequently the elongation of the intestine causes a small bend, with the convexity directed ventrad, to appear in the umbilical region. This bend gradually increases until the gut forms a single long loop, beginning a short distance below the pylorus and directed ventro-caudad. The apex of the loop, to which the vitello-intestinal duct is attached (Fig. 98) (cf.p. 34) projects beyond the abdominal cavity into the hollow of the umbilical cord, constituting the so-called "umbilical or embryonal intestinal hernia." This entrance of the apex of the intestinal umbilical loop into the umbilical cord begins in embryos of about 10 mm. During the succeeding weeks—up to the tenth— the segment of the intestine thus lodged within the hollow of the umbilical cord increases. After this period the intestinal coils are gradually withdrawn within the abdomen. The explanation of this temporary extrusion of the intestine into the umbilical cord is probably to be found in the strain produced by the yolk-sac which is attached by the vitello-intestinal duct to the apex of the umbilical loop. As we have seen (p. 35) the site of the original apex of the loop may still be indicated in the adult by the persistence of a portion of the vitello-intestinal duct as a "Meckel's diverticulum."

In its simplest primitive condition the loop presents a proximal, descending or efferent limb, an apex, and an ascending, returning or afferent limb (Fig. 98). In the human embryo these segments of the loop furnish the jejuno-ileum and portions of the large intestine, in a manner to be subsequently detailed.

This stage in the development of the higher vertebrate intestine is well illustrated by the alimentary tract of the mud-puppy, *Necturus maculatus*, shown in Fig. 99, which represents the entire situs viscerum of an adult female animal.

The stomach is tubular, not distinctly differentiated from the œsophagus, placed vertically in the long axis of the body. The pyloric end is marked by a constriction separating stomach from midgut and immediately beyond this point the pancreas is applied to the intestine. The rest of the intestinal canal forms a simple loop, the descending limb presenting

21

one or two primitive convolutions. There is no marked differentiation between large and small intestine, the canal possessing a nearly uniform caliber from pylorus to cloaca.

2. The differentiation of the small from the large intestine, marked by the appearance of the cæcal bud or protrusion (Fig. 100), takes place in the ascending segment of the umbilical loop a short distance from the apex. In the human embryo the cæcal bud appears in the 6th week as a plainly marked protuberance, which grows very slowly in length and circumference. It shows very early an unequal rate of development; the terminal piece, not keeping pace in growth with the proximal portion, is converted into the vermiform appendix, while the proximal segment develops into the cæcum proper. The increase in the length of the loop, which begins to be marked in the 7th week, is not uniform. The apex is the first portion to present the evidences of this growth. Subsequently the descending limb grows in length very rapidly and is early thrown into numerous coils of the future mobile portion of the small intestine (jejuno-ileum). Even before the withdrawal of the apex of the loop within the abdominal cavity a prominent coil of these convolutions is found protruding in the umbilical region (Fig. 544). The ascending limb of the loop from which a portion of the large intestine is developed, grows comparatively slowly at this time.

FIG. 100.—Schema of human embryonic intestinal canal after differentiation of the large and small intestine.

FIG. 101.—Human embryo of 2.15 mm., twelve days old. Seessel's sac is the cephalic blind termination of the embryonic foregut before the communication with the ectodermal invagination of the stomadæum has been formed. (Reconstruction after His.)

FIG. 102.—Representation of alimentary canal and appendages of human embryo of 4.1 mm.; isolated. × 15. (Kollmann, after His.)

FIG. 103.—Alimentary canal and appendages of human embryo of 12.5 mm. × 12. (Kollmann, after His.)

FIG. 104.—A. Schematic representation of alimentary canal, with umbilical loop and mesenteric attachments in human embryo of about six weeks. B and C, stages in the intestinal rotation.

The future portions of the human adult alimentary tract below the stomach may be referred, in reference to their derivation, to this primitive condition of the tube as follows:

1. The segment of small intestine situated between the pylorus and the beginning or point of departure of the proximal or descending limb of the umbilical loop, develops into the *duodenum*. This portion of the small intestine is indicated early in embryos of 2.15 mm. (Fig. 101), by the origin of the hepatic duct from the intestinal tube. Somewhat later, in embryos of 4.10-5 mm. length, (Fig. 102) it becomes additionally marked by the origin of the pancreatic diverticulum. The duodenum, at first straight, now begins to curve, forming a short *duodenal loop* or *bend*. In embryos of 6 weeks the duodenum forms a simple loop placed transversely below the pyloric extremity of the stomach (Figs. 103 and 104).

2. The descending limb, the apex and a small part of the ascending limb of the umbilical loop form the jejuno-ileum.

3. The remainder of the ascending limb forms the cæcum and appendix, the ascending and transverse colon.

4. The distal straight portion of the primitive tube forms the terminal portion of the transverse colon (the splenic flexure), the descending colon, sigmoid flexure and rectum.

The primitive condition of the embryonal mammalian alimentary tract, after differentiation of the large intestine is well illustrated by some of the lower vertebrates in which development never proceeds beyond this stage. Fig. 112 shows the entire alimentary canal of a teleost fish, the conger eel (*Echelus conger*) isolated.

The preparation forms a good illustration of the embryonal stage of the higher vertebrates in which development has not proceeded beyond the formation of the simple umbilical loop, about corresponding to the schematic Fig. 98. The stomach is differentiated both by its caliber and by the formation of a pyloric ring valve.

The midgut forms a simple loop with a descending and ascending limb closely bound together by mesenteric attachment. Different from the course of development followed in the human embryo is the situation of the ileo-colic junction. The same appears in the terminal straight segment of the canal—corresponding to the human descending colon—

while in the human embryo the differentiation of small and large intestine takes place in the course of the ascending limb of the loop. This condition depends upon the relatively much shorter extent of the teleost endgut compared with the human large intestine. Other examples are afforded by the alimentary tract of some of the Amphibia and Reptilia. Fig. 105 shows the alimentary canal of *Rana catesbiana*, the common bull frog. The stomach, fairly well differentiated, is succeeded by the small intestine of considerable length and uniform caliber. The proximal portion of the small intestine is characterized as duodenum by its connection with liver and pancreas. In the remaining portion of the intestinal canal it is not difficult to recognize the elements of the umbilical loop of the higher mammalian embryo. The larger mass of the jejuno-ileal coils is developed from the descending limb of the loop; a smaller number of convolutions belong to the returning or ascending limb, which also includes the ileo-colic junction. The very short large intestine of the frog passes straight down to enter the cloaca. Another example, in which the early embryonal stages of the higher mammalia are illustrated by the permanent structure of one of the lower vertebrates, is given in Fig. 106, which shows the alimentary tract of a chelonian, *Pseudemys elegans*, the pond turtle. The bilobed liver fits over the well-differentiated stomach in the manner of a saddle. The stomach itself, as in chelonians generally, has a markedly transverse position and passes under cover of the right lobe of the liver into the duodenum. The coils of small intestine form a prominent mass, which, however, when unravelled as shown in the figure, permits us to recognize its identity with the mammalian embryonic umbilical loop. The well-marked ileo-colic junction is situated at the termination of the returning limb of the loop, close to the beginning of the descending limb. This close approximation of the duodenum and colon (duodeno-colic isthmus) forms one of the most important factors in the further development of the mammalian intestinal canal and will again be referred to below.

FIG. 106.—*Pseudemys elegans*, pond turtle. Alimentary canal. (Columbia University Museum, No. 1437.)

FIG. 105.—*Rana catesbiana*, bull-frog. Alimentary canal and appendages. (Columbia University Museum, No. 1454.)

FIG. 107.—Abdominal viscera of *Tamandua bivittata*, the little ant-eater, seen from the left, with the intestines turned to the right. (From a fresh dissection.)

FIG. 108.—The same view, from another specimen. Figures 107 and 108 should be studied and compared together, as each supplements the other.

FIG. 109.—Abdominal viscera of *Tamandua bivittata*, the little ant-eater, seen from the right, with the intestines turned to the left. (From a fresh dissection.)

FIG. 110.—The same view, from another specimen.

FIG. 111.—Schematic representation of the development of the mesentery of the umbilical loop.

FIG. 112.—Alimentary canal, isolated and in section, of *Echelus conger*, the conger eel. (Columbia University Museum, No. 1812.)

FIG. 113.—*Chelydra serpentina*, snapping turtle; intestinal canal, pancreas, and spleen, isolated. (Columbia University Museum, No. 1369)

From the ileo-colic junction the large intestine of the turtle continues caudad to the cloaca in a nearly straight line. The same primitive condition of the intestinal canal may be observed in some members of man's own class, the mammalia—as in certain edentates. Figs. 107 and 108 show the entire abdominal portion of the alimentary tract in *Tamandua bivittata*, the little ant-eater of Brazil. The stomach is turned cephalad and the great omentum elevated. The intestines are turned over to the right side.

It will be observed that in spite of the numerous coils of the small intestine the general arrangement of the alimentary canal corresponds to the primitive scheme shown in Fig. 98. The entire intestinal canal is attached by a continuous vertical mesentery to the dorsal median line of the abdominal cavity ventrad of the vertebral column and aorta. The growth in length of the small intestine has necessitated a corresponding lengthening of the attached border of the mesentery—consequently the membrane presents a pleated or crenated appearance. The cæcum is well developed, the ileo-cæcal junction being situated within the returning limb of the loop, a little distance from the apex.

In Figs. 109 and 110, taken from the same specimens, the entire mass of the small intestines has been turned to the left so as to exhibit the right leaf of the common dorsal mesentery and the mesoduodenum, the latter containing the head of the pancreas. It will be noted that the mesentery, expanding beyond the duodeno-colic isthmus, is common to the small and to the proximal portion of the large intestine, *i. e.*, to those segments of the alimentary canal which are developed from the two limbs of the umbilical loop. Figs. 107-110 should be studied and compared together, as each supplements the others.

It will be observed, in reference to the change from the primitive loop to the subsequent increase in the length of the tube and the resulting arrangement of the mesentery, that three successive stages are to be considered, represented schematically in Fig. 111. In the earliest stage (Fig. 111, I.) the two segments of the loop are of equal length, parallel to one another, the distance between the beginning and termination of the loop (1-2) being maintained throughout its extent. Hence the mesentery is of equal width in all its parts within the loop, only drawn out, *i. e.*, away from the vertebral column, in accordance with the length of the loop. In the next stage (Fig. 111, II.) the increase in the length of the intestine is accompanied by a corresponding widening of the mesentery. The points 1 and 2 are still approximately the same distance apart as in the earlier stage, but the increase in the length of the tube between these points forces the two limbs of the loop to abandon their early parallel course, and to form curved lines with the concavity turned toward the mesenteric attachment. In this condition the mesentery consequently forms a widely expanded membrane framed by the intestine and narrowing between the points 1 and 2 to a neck or isthmus which effects the transition between the expanded segment surrounded by the intestine and the rest of the dorsal primitive mesentery. Finally in the stage represented inFig. 111, III., the increase in the length of the small intestine has reached a point where a single curve is no longer sufficient for the accommodation of the growth. Consequently the tube now appears coiled and convoluted, and the mesentery, as it is attached to the gut, of necessity follows all the twists and appears fluted or pleated in its distal attached portion.

If we now carefully examine the conditions presented by the intestine and mesentery in a form like *Tamandua* (Figs. 107 and 108) we will find that they correspond to the developmental facts thus far considered. The termination of the duodenum (1) and the bend in the colon (2) mark the two points at which in the primitive schema (Fig. 111, I.) the umbilical loop begins and terminates. The proximal of these two points (1) corresponds to the termination of the duodenum, which segment extends from here cephalad to the pyloric extremity of the stomach. The distal point (2) is placed on the colon where the returning limb of the loop resumes the original median vertical course of the large intestine. These two points mark the neck of the loop, which we can describe as the *duodeno-colic neck* or*isthmus.*

The same condition is well shown in the intestinal canal of the snapping turtle (Fig. 113). The duodenum and colon approach each other very closely at the isthmus and between these points the convolutions of the intestine extend in a wide circle. We will find this approximation of duodenum and colon a feature which persists throughout all the later developmental stages of the higher vertebrates and has an important bearing on the final arrangement of the intestinal canal in the human adult.

Further Changes in the Development of the Human Alimentary Canal. Rotation of the Intestine. Formation of the Segments of the Colon. Final Permanent Relations of the Segments of the Intestinal Tube.—The next important stage leading up to the final adult disposition of the intestine in man and the higher mammals is the *rotation* of the portions developed from the two limbs of the primitive loop around an oblique axis drawn from the duodeno-colic isthmus to the apex of the loop. The portion of the large intestine, developed from the ascending limb of the loop, moves in the third month to the middle line, coming into contact with the ventral abdominal wall. From here the large intestine passes, ventrad of the jejuno-ileal coils, toward the cephalic end of the abdominal cavity and lies transversely along the greater curvature of the stomach. The growing coils of the small intestine crowd the colon more and more cephalad. In the fourth month the cæcum turns to the right, coming into contact with the caudal surface of the liver, ventrad of the duodenum, and subsequently reaches the ventral surface of the right kidney. As the result of this rotation the ileo-colic junction, cæcum and succeeding portion of the colon are

24

carried from the original position in the distal and left part of the abdomen cephalad and to the right across the proximal (duodenal) portion of the small intestine, while the coils of the jejuno-ileum, developed from the descending limb and apex of the loop, are turned in the opposite direction, caudad and to the left underneath the preceding (Figs. 114 and 115). This change in the relative position of the parts of the intestinal tract and the resulting altered bearing of the colon tothe duodenum will be best appreciated by considering in the first place the effect of the change on the arrangement of the primitive mesentery and the intestinal vessels, and secondly by repeating actually the rotation in the intestinal tract of a mammal (cat) in which the adult arrangement of the intestine and peritoneum permits us to perform the manipulations and note the result.

FIG. 114A.—Intestinal canal in stage of umbilical loop—before rotation. FIG. 114B.—First stage in rotation, colon crossing duodenum.

FIG. 115A.—Second stage in rotation—rotation of small intestine. FIG. 115B.—Schema of intestinal canal after complete rotation and descent of cæcum.

I. Effect of Rotation on the Disposition of the Primitive Mesentery and on the Relative Position of Duodenum and Colon, and Consequent Arrangement of the Intestinal Blood Vessels.—It will be appreciated that in Fig. 111, representing a profile view of the original arrangement, or in Figs. 107 and 108, showing the intestinal canal of *Tamandua*, the left layer of the primitive mesentery is turned toward the observer. The membrane is seen to pass from the ventral aspect of the vertebral column and aorta, through the narrow neck of the duodeno-colic isthmus, to expand in the manner already indicated toward its intestinal attachment. In the rotation of the intestine the twist takes place at the duodeno-colic neck, carrying, as already stated, the large intestine cephalad and to the right, while the jejuno-ileum is turned in the opposite direction caudad and to the left. During this rotation the duodeno-jejunal angle (Figs. 114, B and 115, A) passes to the left underneath the proximal segment of the colon, which now lies ventrad and to the right of the duodenal portion of the small intestine. The mesenteric peritoneum, occupying the bight of the umbilical loop, will, after the rotation, in the left profile view shown in Fig. 104, A and B, turn its original right leaf toward the beholder, *i. e.*, toward the left, while the original left leaf is turned toward the right.

Observation of the difference in the position of the ileo-colic junction will still further accentuate the change in the relative position of the parts which has been effected by the rotation. In the primitive condition shown in Fig. 104, A, the ileum enters the large intestine from right to left, and the concavity of the cæcal bud turns its crescentic margin ventrad and to the right.

After rotation is accomplished (Fig. 104, B and C, and Fig. 115) the ileo-colic entrance takes place in the opposite direction, from left to right and the cæcum turns its concave margin caudad and to the left.

FIG. 116.—Abdominal viscera of *Tamandua bivittata*, with the intestine rotated to correspond to the development in the human subject. (From a fresh dissection.)

FIG. 117.—The same view as Fig. 116, from another specimen.

Figs. 116 and 117 show the intestinal tract of *Tamandua bivittata* arranged so as to correspond to the human embryonic condition after rotation. The cæcum has been brought up and to the right across the proximal duodenal portion of the small intestine, while the jejuno-ileal coils have been turned down and to the left. The rotation has been accomplished by a twist at the duodeno-colic isthmus, and the original right leaf of the mesentery has become the left and *vice versa*. Comparison with Figs. 107 and 108, representing the condition before rotation in the same animal, will indicate the changes which have been accomplished by imitating the course of development followed in the higher mammals.

Failure of rotation and arrest of development at the primitive stage, with consequent persistent embryonic condition of the mesentery, occurs occasionally in man. Such cases have been reported by W. J. Walsham, in St. Barthol. Hosp. Rep., London, Vol. 16. The following four instances of this condition, taken from the Columbia University museum, will illustrate the disposition of the abdominal contents.

25

Fig. 118 shows the arrangement of the abdominal viscera in an adult female body. Beginning at the pyloric extremity of the stomach the entire course of the duodenum can be overlooked and its continuation into the jejuno-ileal division traced. The small intestines occupy the ventral and right part of the cavity. The ileo-colic junction is placed in the lower left-hand corner of the abdomen and the small intestine enters the large from right to left, the ascending colon is situated to the left of the median line and at its point of transition into the segment representing the transverse colon is connected by several adhesions with the ventral surface of the duodenum. The transverse colon, folded into several coils bound together by adhesion, occupies the upper left portion of the abdomen.

Fig. 119, taken from the same specimen, shows the entire mass of intestines lifted up and turned to the left, exposing the background of the abdominal cavity lined by parietal peritoneum. The duodenum is still entirely free and non-adherent to the parietal peritoneum. The continuity of the mesoduodenum with the jejuno-ileal mesentery is well shown. The primitive right leaf of the mesentery is turned to the observer. This layer after completed rotation would form the left layer of the adult mesentery of the jejuno-ileum.

FIG. 118.—Abdominal viscera of adult human female, in a case of arrested rotation of the intestines. (Columbia University Museum, Study Collection.)

FIG. 119.—The same preparation with the intestinal coils displaced upward and to the left.

Fig. 120 illustrates another instance of the same condition in the adult. In this case the duodenum was coiled twice upon itself and adherent to the prerenal parietal peritoneum.

Fig. 121, presenting the same adhesion of the duodenum, illustrates very perfectly the persistence of the narrow duodeno-colic isthmus in cases of non-rotation, as well as the development of the different segments of the adult tract from the limbs of the embryonal umbilical intestinal loop.

It will be observed that beyond the duodeno-colic isthmus the coils of the jejuno-ileum have resulted from the increase in length of the descending limb, the apex and the proximal part of the ascending or recurrent limb, carrying the ileo-colic junction and cæcum. The remainder of the ascending limb, terminating in the embryonic condition at the splenic flexure by passing into the descending colon, has in the course of further development in this individual produced a straight segment—the misplaced ascending colon—and a convoluted and bent representative of the normal transverse colon.

The same disposition of the large intestine may be noted in the other preparations.

FIG. 120.—Abdominal viscera of adult human male; non-rotation of intestine. (Columbia University Museum, Study Collection.)

FIG. 121.—Abdominal viscera of adult human male; non-rotation of intestine. (Columbia University Museum, Study Collection.)

FIG. 122.—Abdominal viscera of child, two years old; non-rotation of intestine. (Columbia University Museum, Study Collection.)

FIG. 123.—Human fœtus at term; abdominal viscera, hardened in situ; non-rotation of cæcum. (Columbia University Museum, No. 1813.)

Fig. 122 shows an instance of non-rotation observed in the human infant at two years of age.

Fig. 123, taken from a fœtus at term, shows the result of failure to completely rotate in the region of the cæcum and ileo-colic junction. The rest of the large intestine has rotated as usual and assumed the normal position. The terminal ileum, however, passes behind the cæcum and enters the large intestine on its right side; the cæcum is turned upwards and to the right and the appendix lies ventrad of the beginning of the ascending colon. In order to produce the normal arrangement, shown in Fig. 124, taken from another fœtus at term, it would be necessary to turn the cæcum and ileo-colic junction in Fig. 123 through half a circle. The cæcum would then turn upwards and to the left, the ileum entering the large intestine from left to right, and the appendix would be placed behind the cæcum and ileo-colic junction. Figs. 125 and 126 show the normal and abnormal arrangement presented by these two preparations diagrammatically. The instances in which in the adult the ileo-colic entrance is placed on the right side of the large intestine and in which the appendix is situated laterad of the ascending colon unquestionably find their explanation in the failure of the intestine to completely rotate at the ileo-colic junction.

FIGS. 125, 126.—Schematic representation of final stages in rotation of cæcum and large intestine.

FIG. 124.—Human fœtus at term; abdominal viscera, hardened *in situ*; normal position of completely rotated cæcum and appendix. (Columbia University Museum, No. 1814.)

FIG. 125.—Just before final rotation of cæcum and terminal ileum. Concavity of cæcum directed cephalad and to right. Terminal ileum enters colon from right to left.

FIG. 126.— Rotation completed. Concavity of cæcum turns caudad and to left. Terminal ileum enters colon from left to right.

FIG. 127.—Adult human subject with non-rotated cæcum. The terminal ileum turns caudad from right to left to enter right side of colon.

FIG. 128.—Adult human subject with non-rotated cæcum, the ileum entering large intestine from the right and behind, and the appendix placed to the right of the ascending colon. (From a fresh dissection.)

The resulting conditions are shown in Figs. 127 and 128, taken from adult human subjects in which the final stage of rotation of the large intestine has not taken place.

In Fig. 127 the terminal ileum is sharply bent on itself and adherent to the prerenal parietal peritoneum. It passes from right to left and downwards to enter the right posterior circumference of the large intestine. The cæcum is turned cephalad and the appendix is in contact with the right lobe of the liver. The cæcum passes with a sharp bend into the obliquely directed ascending colon.

In Fig. 128 the ileum enters the colon from the right and below. The apex of the cæcum is turned cephalad and to the right and the appendix extends beneath peritoneal adhesions along the lateral border of the proximal segment of the colon.

In the next place it is desirable to clearly understand the vascular supply of the intestine before and after rotation and the final relation of the superior mesenteric artery to the transverse portion of the duodenum.

Development of Aortal Arterial System.

The thoracic and abdominal aortæ are at first double, the first aortic arches continuing as so-called "primitive aortæ" ventrad of the vertebral column to the caudal end of the body.

The cephalic portions of the two vessels unite in the chick on the third day and from this point fusion into a single vessel proceeds slowly caudad.

In the rabbit the fusion of the primitive aortæ begins on the ninth day in the region of the lung-buds and progresses from here caudad until by the sixteenth day a single aorta is formed (Fig. 129).

FIG. 129.—Diagrams illustrating the arrangement of the primitive heart and aortic arches. (After Heisler, modified from Allen Thompson.)

That the entire descending aorta in man results from the fusion of two vessels is shown by the rare cases in which the aorta is divided throughout its entire length by a septum.

The arteries of the allantois are originally the terminations of the primitive aortæ. After fusion of the primitive aortæ to form the abdominal aorta the allantoic arteries, now passing as the umbilical arteries to the placenta, appear as the branches of bifurcation of the abdominal aorta, in the same way as the common iliacs do in the adult.

They furnish branches, which at first are very small, to the budding posterior extremities and the pelvic viscera. In time these rudiments of the future external and internal iliac arteries become larger, but as the umbilical arteries continue to develop throughout the entire intra-uterine period they appear even in the fœtus at term as end branches of the aorta, a condition which is only changed after birth by the obliteration of the umbilical

27

arteries and their conversion into the lateral ligaments of the bladder, while the iliac vessels now appear as the terminal aortic branches. The statement that the umbilical arteries appear as the terminal branches of the embryonal aorta requires to be modified in the following respect:

When the allantois develops its arteries are in fact end-branches of the two primitive aortæ. After their fusion and after the formation of the single aorta this vessel is continued beyond the umbilical arteries as a small trunk, the caudal artery or rudiment of the adult sacralis media. Consequently the umbilical arteries are really lateral branches of a median vessel, viz., aorta abdominalis and arteria sacralis media. But as the umbilical vessels are very large and the caudal aorta very small, the former, even under these conditions, appear as the real terminal branches of the abdominal aorta.

The arteries supplying the yolk-sac and subsequently the intestinal canal are the vitelline or omphalo-mesenteric. At first they are branches derived from the two primitive aortæ, and after the fusion of these vessels they arise from the resulting single abdominal aorta. The omphalo-mesenteric arteries are at first multiple and later are reduced to two. When the primitive intestine loses its original close contact with the vertebral column and the common dorsal mesentery develops, the two omphalo-mesenteric arteries unite to form a single vessel, running between the layers of the mesentery. After a short course this artery divides again into two branches, passing one on each side, around the intestinal tube, which has in the meanwhile become closed. Ventrad of the intestine these branches reunite so that the gut is surrounded by a vascular circle. The left half of this loop becomes obliterated and the trunk of the omphalo-mesenteric artery now passes on the right side of the intestine to the umbilicus. The peripheral segment of the omphalo-mesenteric artery disappears with the cessation of the vitelline circulation. The proximal portion, situated between the layers of the mesentery, gives numerous anastomosing branches to the intestine and is converted into the main trunk of the superior mesenteric artery.

The derivation of the superior mesenteric as the fully developed proximal segment of the embryonic omphalo-mesenteric artery passing to the yolk-sac is responsible for the rare anomaly in the adult of a branch of the superior mesenteric artery continuing beyond the intestine to the umbilicus. I have encountered one instance of this persistence of the intra-abdominal portion of the omphalo-mesenteric artery in a male subject 54 years of age. Aconnective strand, containing a small artery derived from the superior mesenteric vessels, extended between the right layer of the mesentery, some distance from its attached border, and the ventral abdominal wall at the umbilicus. The vessel which was pervious throughout, was the size of one of the digital arteries.

Hyrtl has observed the same variation. An example of partial persistence of the omphalo-mesenteric artery in the adult is well seen in the case of Meckel's diverticulum shown inFig. 37, where the arterial vessel continued upon the diverticulum represents the embryonic omphalo-mesenteric artery.

The remaining intestinal arteries are at first more numerous and paired. In man and most mammals they are early reduced in number, passing from the abdominal aorta to the dorsal or attached border of the intestine, between the two peritoneal layers of the primitive dorsal mesentery (Fig. 104). The arterial blood supply of the intestinal canal then presents three general divisions:

1. Vessels pass from the proximal part of the abdominal aorta to the stomach and pyloric portion of the duodenum. This set of vessels forms the rudiment of the future cœliac axis. With the development of the liver and pancreas by budding from the duodenum, and with the appearance of the spleen in the mesoderm of the dorsal mesentery, branches corresponding to these organs (hepatic and splenic arteries) are added to the gastric and duodenal vessels and the adult arrangement of the cœliac axis is thus obtained (Figs. 130, 131, 132 and 133).

FIG. 130.—Diagrammatic representation of the arteries proceeding to the alimentary canal and appendages

FIG. 131.—Diagrammatic representation of the arteries of the alimentary canal in the first stage of intestinal rotation, showing relation of superior mesenteric artery

prior to rotation of intestine (stage of   to the transverse portion of the duodenum.
simple umbilical loop).

FIG. 132.—Arteries   of   FIG. 133.—Final arrangement of arteries of
alimentary canal in the later stages of alimentary canal after completed rotation of the
intestinal rotation.   intestines.

These vessels have an important bearing on the formation of the adult peritoneal
cavity in the retro-gastric space, and will be considered in detail below with that portion of
the subject.

2. The next vessel in order derived from the aorta and supplying the duodenum,
pancreas, the small and a part of the large intestine is the above-mentioned superior
mesenteric artery, which arises from the aorta a short distance caudad of the cœliac axis
(Figs. 130, 131, 132 and 133).

At the time when the intestine still presents the primitive arrangement of the
umbilical loop (Figs. 104 and 130) this vessel passes between the layers of the dorsal
mesentery through the narrow duodeno-colic neck to reach the two limbs and the apex of
the intestinal loop. In its course it gives off successively branches to the gut from each side.
Those from the right side of the main vessel pass to the duodenum, pancreas, jejunum and
ileum. Those from the left side of the main vessel accede in succession to the colic angle of
the isthmus, the proximal portion of the colon, the cæcum and the ileo-colic junction. The
terminal portion of the superior mesenteric artery supplies the ileum near the ileo-colic
entrance. After rotation it will be found that the turn has occurred at the point X (Fig.
130), $i.\ e.$, in that part of the vessel which occupies the duodeno-colic isthmus. Hence it will
be found that the first branches derived from the right side of the primitive superior
mesenteric artery, supplying the duodenum and pancreas (Art. pancreatico-duodenalis
inferior) still arise after rotation from the right side. They are succeeded, beyond the point X,
by the original highest *left* branches passing to colon, cæcum and ileo-colic junction, while all
the original right-sided vessels, except the inferior pancreatico-duodenal, appear now as
branches from the left side of the main artery, supplying the coils of the jejuno-ileum. Hence
in the adult (Fig. 133) the succession of branches derived from the right or concave side of
the superior mesenteric artery is as follows:

FIG. 134.—Schematic representation of intestinal arterial supply from superior
mesenteric artery in cases of arrested rotation of the intestine.

1.	Arteria	pancreatico-duodenalis	inferior.
2.	Arteria	colica	media.
3.	Arteria	colica	dextra.

4. Arteria ileo-colica.

On the other hand, the first branches from what has now become the left or convex
side of the vessel are the original lower right-hand vessels to the small intestine developed
from the descending limb of the loop. Hence in the adult the left side of the superior
mesenteric vessel gives rise to the vasa intestini tenuis.

3. The caudal intestinal arterial branch derived from the aorta is the inferior
mesenteric artery supplying parts of the transverse colon, the descending colon, sigmoid
flexure and rectum (Figs. 130, 131, 132, and 133).

On the other hand in the cases of non-rotation of the intestine as above described
in Figs. 118-122, the embryonic type of the intestinal arterial supply persists, as indicated
schematically in Fig. 134. Not only the pancreatico-duodenalis inferior, but all the remaining
branches to the small intestine are derived from the right side of the superior mesenteric
artery. The terminal branches of the main artery supply the ileo-colic junction, while the
arterial supply of the large intestine, A. colica dextra and media, are given off from the left
side of the parent vessel.

II. **Demonstration of Intestinal Rotation in the Cat.**—The changes in the relative
position of the different intestinal segments and the final disposition of the mesenteries and
blood vessels can best be understood by the direct examination of the abdominal contents in
an animal whose permanent adult arrangement corresponds to one of the early embryonal

29

human stages, and in which the necessary manipulations can readily be carried out and their results noted.

It is doubtful if the above detailed developmental stages in man can ever be clearly comprehended unless the student will for himself examine the conditions and perform the manipulations in one of the lower mammals.

The necessity of keeping the three dimensions of space in mind and the fact that certain structures during and after rotation cover and obscure each other, make diagrams and drawings unsatisfactory unless the actual examination of the object itself is combined with their study. Fortunately, among the common domestic animals of convenient size easily obtained the cat answers every purpose of this study admirably. The student is earnestly urged to pursue his study of the development and adult arrangement of the human abdominal viscera and peritoneum in the light which the anatomy of this animal can shed on the complicated and obscure conditions encountered in the human subject. The plan of having the opened abdominal cavity of the cat directly side by side with the human subject, while the arrangement of the abdominal viscera and peritoneum is considered, cannot be recommended too highly.

DIRECTIONS.—After killing the animal with chloroform the abdominal cavity is to be freely opened by a cruciform incision and the skin flaps turned well back and secured in this position. It is well to select a male animal or an unimpregnated female, as the size of the pregnant uterus in the later stages renders the examination of the abdominal viscera and peritoneum more difficult.

FIG. 135.—Abdominal viscera of cat; great omentum raised; intestines turned down and to left. (From a fresh dissection.)

For purposes of careful study and comparison of the vascular relations of the abdomen, it is highly desirable to inject the animal with differently colored gelatine, starch or plaster of Paris mass. The arterial injection can be made through the carotid artery, the systemic venous injection through the femoral vein, and the portal circulation can be filled after opening the abdomen, by injection through the superior mesenteric or splenic veins. Animals prepared in this manner are especially useful for the study of the upper portion of the abdominal cavity and of the peritoneal relations of liver, stomach, spleen, pancreas and duodenum. They may be kept for permanent reference in a 5 per cent. solution of formaline or 50 per cent. alcohol.

After opening the abdominal cavity turn the great omentum up over the ventral surface of the thorax and secure it in this position, thus exposing the underlying intestines completely (Fig. 135). Trace in the first place the entire course of the intestinal tube from the pyloric extremity of the stomach down. It will be noticed that the first portion of the small intestine (duodenum) is freely movable, completely invested by peritoneum and attached to the dorsal midline by a mesoduodenum between the layers of which a portion of the pancreas is seen.

Following the duodenum caudad it will be observed that the gut can be traced directly continuous with the remaining coils of the small intestine. The ileo-colic junction and the beginning of the large intestine are marked by a short pointed cæcum. The large intestine is short, as it is in all carnivore mammals, and passes from the cæcum almost directly down into the pelvis.

Take the cæcum and the first portion of the large intestine and turn them caudad and over to the left side as far as the peritoneal connections will permit.

Spread out the coils of the small intestine in the opposite direction, i. e., over to the right side.

The arrangement of the intestinal tract after these manipulations should appear as shown inFigs. 136 and 137.

FIG. 136.—Abdominal viscera of cat, hardened; omentum removed to display derivation of intestines from umbilical loop and the relation of the superior mesenteric artery and common dorsal mesentery to the small and large intestines. (Columbia University Museum, No 728.)

FIG. 137.—Abdominal cavity of cat. (From a fresh dissection.)

30

It will be seen that all the essential features described for the corresponding stage in the human embryo (Fig. 104, *A*) exist here. The proximal portion of the small intestine (duodenum) retains its freedom and mobility, being attached to the ventral surface of the vertebral column by the portion of the primitive mesentery which now constitutes the mesoduodenum. The gut itself forms a bend with the convexity turned to the right.

Observe in the next place that the point (Fig. 136, *X*), where small intestine and colon approach each other closely, marks the situation of the fœtal duodeno-colic isthmus. The small intestine at this point corresponds to the future duodeno-jejunal angle as will be seen after rotation has been accomplished.

Recalling the development of the jejuno-ileum it will not be difficult to recognize in the numerous coils of small intestine which succeed to the duodeno-colic isthmus the results of the increase in length of the descending or efferent limb of the human embryonal umbilical loop. Tracing these coils it will be found that the terminal portions of the ileum correspond to the apex and to the proximal part of the ascending or recurrent limb of the primitive loop, while the remainder of this limb furnishes the cæcum and the next succeeding segment of the large intestine. Following the tube up to this point the colic boundary of the duodeno-colic isthmus will be reached; from here the short large intestine of the carnivore descends straight into the pelvis, attached to the ventral surface of the vertebral column by a mesocolon which corresponds to the distal part of the original primitive dorsal mesentery.

Now with the parts still in this position examine carefully the arrangement of the mesentery and of the intestinal blood vessels. Starting with the duodenum it will be seen that the primitive sagittal mesentery of this portion of the intestine has followed the gut in its turn to the right, so that the original right layer of the sagittal membrane is now directed dorsad and lies in contact with the parietal peritoneum which invests the background of the abdominal cavity in the right lumbar region below the liver and covers the ventral surface of the right kidney. Beneath this parietal peritoneum the inferior vena cava is seen, receiving the right renal vein and ascending to enter the dorso-caudal aspect of the right lobe of the liver. If now we assume that in the cat the opposed serous surfaces of the original right leaf of the mesoduodenum, now directed dorsad, and of the parietal peritoneum adhere to each other, and that the visceral peritoneum covering the dorsal surface of the descending duodenum likewise becomes obliterated by adhesion to the subjacent parietal peritoneum, we will obtain the arrangement found in the adult human subject, in which the descending duodenum is fixed by adhesion below the right lobe of the liver and ventrad of the medial portion of right kidney, right renal vein and inferior vena cava. During this process of anchoring the head of the pancreas, which is found between the two layers of the free mesoduodenum of the cat, would also become fixed to the abdominal background by adhesion of the original right leaf of the mesoduodenum, investing what has now become the dorsal surface of the pancreas, to the parietal peritoneum. The original left layer of the primitive mesoduodenum would then appear as *secondary* parietal peritoneum covering what has now become the ventral surface of the transversely disposed head of the gland. The stages may be represented schematically in Figs. 138-140.

FIGS. 138-140.—Diagrammatic representation of three stages in the development of the mesoduodenum, duodenum, and pancreas leading to the secondary "retroperitoneal" position of these viscera.

FIG. 138.—Free mesoduodenum in sagittal plane, including head of pancreas between right and left layers.

FIG. 139.—Mesoduodenum folded to right; left leaf has become ventral; right dorsal, directed toward primitive prerenal parietal peritoneum.

FIG. 140.—Fixation of head of pancreas and duodenum under cover of secondary parietal peritoneum by adhesion of apposed surfaces of mesoduodenum and primitive parietal peritoneum.

Figs. 138 and 139 shows the arrangement in the cat where a free duodenum and mesoduodenum exists, with the pancreas included between its layers.[2]

It will be noticed that the duodenum in the cat can be carried over to the median line (Fig. 138) exposing the entire ventral aspect of the right kidney and the inferior vena cava beneath the primary lumbar parietal peritoneum. This manipulation will also expose the dorsal surface of the head of the pancreas, covered by what originally was the right leaf of the mesoduodenum.

Fig. 140 indicates the results of adhesion of the duodenum, pancreas and mesoduodenum to the parietal peritoneum as it normally occurs in the human subject. It will be seen that the primary parietal peritoneum can be traced mesad over the ventral surface of the right kidney as far as the point X, and that from here on to the median line the peritoneum is *secondary*parietal peritoneum, consisting of the visceral peritoneal investment of the ventral surface of the duodenum and of the original left leaf of the mesoduodenum, beneath which the ventral surface of the pancreas is seen. Pancreas and duodenum occupy in the adult secondarily a "retro-peritoneal" position, *i. e.*, the peritoneum now covering the ventral surface of these viscera appears as a continuation of the parietal peritoneum, the transition between primary and secondary parietal peritoneum occurring along the line marked X in Fig. 140. The opposed peritoneal surfaces indicated by the dotted lines have become adherent and converted into loose connective tissue in which the pancreas and duodenum lie imbedded. In the human embryo this process of adhesion begins in the eighth week, starting at the duodeno-jejunal flexure and ascending gradually toward the pylorus. At the end of the fourth month the union is complete.

Proceeding caudad it will next be observed that the peritoneum of the mesentery occupies the narrow neck of the duodeno-colic isthmus, and that large vessels (the superior mesenteric) pass between its two layers at this point to supply the segments of the intestine forming the loop. In conformity with the greatly increased length of the intestine it will be found that the mesentery expands from the narrow pedicle at the neck in a fan-shaped manner in order to develop a sufficiently long margin for attachment to the intestine. The following points should be carefully borne in mind in studying the mesentery with the intestines in this position:

1. The mesentery presents two free surfaces, right and left. With the coils of the small intestine turned over to the right, the left leaf of the mesentery is turned toward the observer.

FIG. 141.—Schematic representation of mesentery of umbilical loop, common to small intestine and proximal portion of large intestine.

2. Inasmuch as the descending limb of the embryonic loop has developed the greater part of the small intestine, while a portion of the large intestine (cæcum and colon up to the isthmus) is the result of differentiation within the ascending or returning limb of the loop, it will be at once apparent that the double peritoneal layer which extends between the duodeno-colic isthmus and the attached border of the gut is partly mesentery of the small intestine, partly mesocolon passing to the large intestine (cæcum and proximal colon). This condition may be indicated schematically in Fig. 141.

The curved line A may be taken as an arbitrary division between the portion of the membrane which on the right of the figure passes to the small intestine, and the portion which proceeds to the left to be attached to the large intestine. In other words the line will schematically separate the true mesenteric from the mesocolic segment of the primitive membrane.

With the parts in their present position this line might be assumed to indicate a strip along which the opposed serous surfaces of the parietal peritoneum and the right leaf of the primitive mesentery became adherent. In that case an actual division into a mesenteric and mesocolic segment would have been effected.

Ventrad and to the right of this line of adhesion we would trace that portion of the primitive membrane which now passes to the coils of the small intestine as the true mesentery, having an apparent origin in the background of the abdomen to the dotted line of adhesion. In the same manner the peritoneal layers passing to the left to reach the cæcum and beginning of the colon would appear as a free mesocolon with the same line of apparent origin from the background of the abdomen. (cf. p. 80.)

These considerations should be followed out in the dissection of the cat in order to become familiar with the principle of *secondary lines of origin* for peritoneal layers. As we will see later this factor is of importance in correctly estimating the value of the human adult conditions.

3. A brief consideration of the mechanical conditions and comparison with the earlier stages will show why the peritoneal layers which occupy the bight of the fully developed umbilical loop are especially prone to develop secondary lines and areas of adhesion to other serous surfaces. If we compare the dorsal mesentery in its primitive condition, before the straight intestinal tube has become differentiated into the subsequent segments, and before the umbilical loop has been formed (Fig. 142), with the later stages represented by the intestines of the cat as now arranged (Figs. 143 and 144), it will be seen that the vertical line of attachment to the ventral surface of the vertebral column, between the points *a* and *b* corresponds in the advanced stages to the interval *ab* separating the two points of the duodeno-colic isthmus; also that the entire mesenteric peritoneal surface beyond the isthmus is the result of drawing out and lengthening the intestinal tract. Consequently folding or overlapping of this extensive membrane affords opportunities for adhesions between its own serous surfaces or between it and the remaining visceral and parietal peritoneum of the abdomen.

FIGS. 142-144.—Schematic representation of three stages in the development of the mesentery of the umbilical intestinal loop.

FIG. 142.—Early stage before differentiation of intestinal canal.

FIG. 143.—Stage of umbilical loop. Differentiation of common dorsal mesentery of earlier stage into dorsal mesogastrium, mesoduodenum, primitive mesentery of umbilical loop, and descending mesocolon.

FIG. 144.—Final stage. With complete differentiation of large and small intestine, the primitive mesentery of the umbilical loop contains not only the mesentery of the future jejuno-ileum, but also the mesocola and the ascending and transverse colon, developed from the ascending or afferent limb of the umbilical loop.

FIG. 145.—Abdominal viscera of cat, with intestines rotated to correspond to the stage in the development of the human canal in which the cæcum has reached the subhepatic position, but before the establishment of the ascending colon. (From a fresh dissection.)

Moreover, it will be appreciated that the entire extensive coil of intestines extending between the two boundaries of the duodeno-colic isthmus (*a, b*) is suspended from the back part of the abdomen by a narrow pedicle and that consequently rotation will readily occur around the axis drawn through the neck of the isthmus.

Now proceed to illustrate on the cat the result of the rotation as it occurs normally during the development of the primate intestinal tract. Take the cæcum and commencement of the colon and draw the same over to the right across the duodeno-colic isthmus and the duodenum. Twist or rotate the entire mass of small intestines around the isthmic pedicle, so that the original left leaf of the mesentery will look to the right and *vice versa* (Fig. 145). The conditions thus established will be found to correspond to the schemata shown in Figs. 114 and 115. The main features of the intestinal tract in the rearranged position will be as follows:

1. The two points, *a* and *b*, of the duodeno-colic isthmus (Fig. 145) are still close together, but reversed in position, *b* is in front and to the right, *a* behind and to the left, whereas before the rotation *b* was situated below and to the left, *a* above and to the right (Fig. 135).

2. The direction of the ileo-colic entrance is reversed, the ileum now entering the large intestine from below and the left upwards and to the right, instead of from right to left.

3. The descending duodenum is now situated dorsad to the colon.

4. The original left leaf of the mesentery has become the right, and *vice versa*.

5. The superior mesenteric artery crosses over the transverse portion of the duodenum, and with the exception of the inferior pancreatico-duodenal artery the original right-sided branches now arise from the left side of the vessel and *vice versa*.

It is now time to compare the conditions established in the cat by the manipulations just detailed with the arrangement of the adult human intestinal tract and peritoneum below the level of the transverse colon and mesocolon.

I. The shortness of the large intestine in the cat will require careful manipulation in order to produce a disposition in conformity with the arrangement of this portion of the human intestinal tract. By stretching the gut somewhat and pulling it well out of the pelvis sufficient length will be obtained to establish an ascending, transverse and descending colon. Move the cæcum from the subhepatic position which it occupies immediately after rotation (Fig. 145) down to the lower and right-hand corner of the abdomen. Pull the distal portion of the large intestine well out of the pelvis and obtain thus sufficient length to establish an ascending, transverse and descending division each provided with a free mesocolon (Fig. 146). In the formation of the three definite main segments of the human large intestine, ascending, transverse and descending colon, the following stages may be recognized:

FIG. 146.—Abdominal viscera of cat, with the intestines rotated to correspond to the adult human disposition, with ascending, transverse, and descending segments of the colon. (From a fresh dissection.)

FIG. 147.—Human fœtus, 6.6 cm., vertex-coccygeal measure; liver removed. (Columbia University Museum, Study Collection.) × 4.

1. Immediately after rotation the large intestine lies transversely along the greater curvature of the stomach, with the cæcum on the right side in front of the duodenum and closely applied to the caudal surface of the right lobe of the liver (Fig. 147).

PERSISTENCE OF SUBHEPATIC POSITION OF CÆCUM IN ADULT.—The period at which the cæcum descends into the iliac fossa is liable to a considerable range of variation.

Treves found in two fœtus, measuring respectively 4½" and 5½", the cæcum on a level with the caudal end of the right kidney, while in several individuals at full term the caput coli was still placed immediately below the liver, with no large intestine in the place of the ascending colon. This condition is well illustrated in the fœtus shown in Fig. 124.

The cæcum may remain undescended throughout life. Treves, in an examination of 100 bodies, found this condition in two subjects, both females, one 41, the other 74 years of age. Both cases presented an identical disposition. There was no large intestine in the place of the ascending colon. The cæcum was placed on the right side, immediately underneath the liver, just to the right of the gall-bladder; it was quite horizontal in position, continuing the long axis of the transverse colon and included between the layers of the transverse mesocolon. From the extremity of the cæcum a horizontal fold was continued to the abdominal parietes and upon it the edge of the liver rested. In one of these instances the colon from the tip of the cæcum to the splenic flexure measured 38". The great omentum was attached only to the left half of this portion. The descending colon was very long, measuring 15".

In the other case the distance from the tip of the cæcum to the splenic flexure was 27", the great omentum commencing 5" from the former point. The descending colon was of normal length.

In both bodies the remaining viscera were normal.

2. The cæcum next descends ventrad of right kidney to the iliac fossa. The future ascending colon is at this time placed very obliquely on account of the large size of the fœtal liver, and passes without a marked angle into the transverse segment. Thus in Fig. 148, from a fœtus 5" in length, the descending colon is vertical and the splenic flexure well marked, forming the highest point of the colic arch. There is no hepatic flexure, and no ascending and transverse colon, but instead of these an oblique segment passing upwards and to the left between cæcum and splenic flexure.

This disposition, due to the large size of the liver, is still marked at times in the fœtus at term, and occasionally even in children up to 2 or 3 years of age.

FIG. 148.—Abdominal viscera of

FIG. 149.—Abdominal viscera of human fœtus at term, hardened *in situ*; hepatic flexure formed and ascending and

34

human fœtus of 12.5 cm., vertex-coccygeal measure, hardened *in situ*; transverse and ascending colon not yet differentiated. (Columbia University Museum, No. 1815.) Natural size.

transverse colon differentiated. (Columbia University Museum, No. 1816.)

3. The ascending colon is subsequently differentiated from the transverse segment and the hepatic flexure formed consequent upon the diminution of the relative size of the liver, which permits the fœtal oblique segment of the colon extending in the earlier stages between the right iliac fossa and the spleen to become divided by a right-angled (hepatic) bend or flexure into an ascending and a transverse segment (Fig. 149).

4. The splenic flexure develops early and is well marked. It indicates the point of transition of the original ascending limb of the umbilical loop into the remaining vertical median segment of the large intestine, from which the descending colon is formed.

In the adult the ascending and descending portions of the colon are vertical. The transverse colon is not quite horizontal since the splenic flexure is higher and placed more dorsally than the hepatic flexure. In the embryo the rapidly-growing coils of the small intestine push the descending colon to the left and dorsad into close contact with the dorsal abdominal wall.

FIG. 150.—Caudal portion of human embryo of 5 mm., with the end- and caudal gut at the highest stage of its development. × 25. (Reconstruction after His.)

A small bend which appears about the middle of the third month in the left iliac fossa indicates the rudiment of the future sigmoid flexure or omega loop.

The rest of the endgut follows the body wall in a well-marked curve, whose termination lies within the concavity of the caudal portion of the embryo (Fig. 150). From this terminal part the rectum develops after the division of the cloaca and the union of the proctodæum with the entodermal intestinal pouch has taken place as detailed above.

The early position of the colon produced by the large size of the fœtal liver, and before the descent of the cæcum has occurred, is shown in Fig. 124. In Fig. 123, where the liver has regained its normal proportions with reference to the abdominal cavity and viscera, and the cæcum has descended into the right iliac fossa, the hepatic flexure is well marked and the first segment of the colon has acquired the vertical position on the right side, the single obliquely transverse segment of Fig. 124, having become divided into an ascending and a transverse colon.

[Fig. 124. Early stage. Liver relatively large. Proximal portion of the colon extends obliquely between the right lumbar region and the spleen. The cæcum has not yet descended.

Fig. 123. Later stage. The cæcum occupies the right iliac fossa. Relative reduction in the size of the liver allows the colic segment to be divided by the hepatic flexure into an ascending colon and a transverse colon.]

FIG. 151.—Abdominal viscera of *Macacus rhesus*, rhesus monkey, hardened in situ. (Columbia University Museum, No. 1817.)

At times the transverse colon, whose normal average length in the adult is 20″, greatly exceeds this measurement and forms an arch which hangs down or makes a well-marked V-shaped bend with the apex directed toward the pubes. This is the normal arrangement of this portion of the large intestine in many of the lower primates. Fig. 151 shows the abdominal viscera of *Macacus rhesus*, hardened *in situ*, seen from the front and the right side, with the omentum turned up over the stomach. The transverse colon forms an extensive V-shaped bend, whose apex reaches to the pubes, from which point the large intestine turns again cephalad and dorsad to form the splenic flexure and then descends to the pelvis.

The average length of the ascending colon in the adult, measured from the tip of the cæcum to the hepatic flexure, was found by Treves in his series of 100 bodies to be 8″, while the descending colon, from the splenic flexure to the beginning of the sigmoid loop, measured 8½″.

The descending colon may at times be much longer, up to 15″, and become convoluted.

II. In the next place, in order to understand the arrangement of the peritoneum in this lower larger compartment of the abdomen, disregard for the present the peritoneal connections of the stomach, liver, pancreas and spleen, and the folds of the great omentum entirely. This latter membrane is adherent in the adult human subject by its dorsal surface to the upper margin of the transverse colon, so that in turning the omentum up over the ventral chest wall the transverse colon will be carried with the omentum and the lower layer of the transverse mesocolon will be put upon the stretch. This membrane forms in adult man by its transverse attachment to the abdominal background the cephalic limit of the larger lower compartment of the abdomen, which is framed laterally by ascending and descending colon, continuous below with the pelvic cavity and occupied chiefly by the freely movable coils of the jejuno-ileum.

Remember that the duodenum starting from the pyloric extremity of the stomach first turns cephalad and dorsad in contact with the caudal surface of the right lobe of the liver, forming the first portion or hepatic angle of the duodenum; that in the next place the second or descending portion of the duodenum passes down in front of the medial part of the ventral surface of the right kidney and the inferior vena cava, but *behind* the right extremity (hepatic flexure) of what after rotation and formation of the ascending colon appears as the transverse colon; that consequently the descending duodenum is divided by its intersection with the transverse colon into a cephalic supra-colic and a caudal infra-colic segment.

Also remember that the second angle of the duodenum (transition between the descending and transverse portions) is consequently situated to the right of the vertebral column below the level of the transverse colon and the secondary attachment presently to be considered of the transverse mesocolon to the background of the abdominal cavity.

The third portion of the duodenum extends from this point more or less transversely—depending upon the type—to the left, across the vertebral column and aorta. This transverse portion, after the rotation of the primitive loop at the duodeno-colic angle, is crossed in the direction caudad and ventrad by the superior mesenteric vessels, which hence divide this portion of the intestine into a right and left segment.

The latter turns cephalad and ventrad on the left side of the vertebral column (4th or ascending portion) to become continuous at the duodeno-jejunal angle with the free or floating small intestine (jejunum).

If we imagine in the cat the duodenum anchored or fixed by adhesion of the dorsal (originally right) leaf of the mesoduodenum and of its own dorsal visceral peritoneum to the abdominal parietal peritoneum in the manner above indicated (p. 70) as far as the duodeno-jejunal angle we will have conditions established which correspond to those found in the human adult abdominal cavity.

III. It is next necessary to study carefully the disposition of the primitive dorsal mesentery connected after rotation with the different segments of the intestinal tube, ascending, transverse and descending colon and free small intestine.

In order to obtain in the cat a cephalic limit to the region now under consideration which will correspond to the arrangement of the adult human peritoneum, we will begin with the peritoneal membrane attached to the portion of the colon which in the rearranged intestinal tract represents the human transverse colon. This transverse segment of the large intestine is now made to extend directly across the abdomen from the liver to the spleen. The two layers composing the transverse mesocolon are an upper or cephalic and a lower or caudal layer.

Now it will be seen in the cat that the upper or cephalic layer of the transverse mesocolon thus established is continuous on each side with the dorsal (originally right) leaf of the ascending and with the dorsal (originally left) leaf of the descending mesocolon, which peritoneal layers are in direct opposition to the parietal lumbar and prerenal peritoneum. On the other hand, the inferior or ventral layer of the transverse mesocolon is continuous on each side of the median line with the ventral (originally respectively left and right) leaves of the same mesocola, while at the site of the duodeno-colic isthmus the two layers of the transverse mesocolon are continuous as originally with the two layers of the mesentery of the jejuno-ileum (Fig. 146).

36

FIGS. 152-154.—Schematic representation of peritoneum in fixation of descending duodenum and formation of transverse colon and mesocolon.

FIG. 152.—Sagittal section through right kidney and descending duodenum before adhesion of latter to parietal peritoneum.

FIG. 153.—Adhesion of descending duodenum to primitive parietal peritoneum. Colon and mesocolon after rotation of the intestine, but before adhesion.

FIG. 154.—Adhesion of mesocolon to duodenum and primitive parietal peritoneum, resulting in formation of root of transverse mesocolon.

Now fix the transverse mesocolon firmly against the background of the abdomen and place the ascending and descending colon as far as possible over to the right and left side respectively. We will assume a line of secondary adhesion between the transverse mesocolon and the parietal peritoneum investing the dorsal abdominal wall. Along this line the upper or cephalic surface of the transverse mesocolon would become continuous with the dorsal parietal peritoneum, while the lower or caudal layer would still be continuous with the left leaf of the ascending and the right leaf of the descending mesocolon. We have already seen that the duodenum and mesoduodenum become anchored in the subhepatic region and that the visceral ventral peritoneum of the gut and the original left leaf of the mesoduodenum appear then as secondary parietal peritoneum. Hence a sagittal section through the right lumbar region, right kidney and descending duodenum would, immediately after rotation and establishment of the transverse mesocolon, show the peritoneal arrangement indicated in Fig. 153. After adhesion of the transverse mesocolon continuity would be established between its upper or cephalic layer and the secondary parietal peritoneum investing the supra-colic portion of the descending duodenum (Fig. 154) while its caudal layer becomes continuous with the secondary parietal peritoneum covering the infra-colic segment of the duodenum and the lower portion of the ventral surface of the right kidney.

Reference to the schematic Figs. 152, 153 and 154, will show that the adult duodenum becomes fixed to the posterior parietes of the abdomen by adhesion of its visceral serous covering and of the dorsal layer of the mesoduodenum to the primitive parietal peritoneum. The supra-colic segment of the adult descending duodenum lies under cover of a single peritoneal layer, derived from its own visceral investment and appearing as secondary parietal peritoneum by continuity laterad along the line of adhesion with the primitive parietal peritoneum covering the upper part of ventral surface of right kidney, while mesad, the layer covering this segment of the duodenum, is continued into the secondary parietal peritoneum derived from the left or ventral leaf of the mesoduodenum and covering the ventral surface of the pancreas (cf. Figs. 138-140).

On the other hand, the infra-colic segment of the descending duodenum, as well as the lower and mesal angle of the ventral surface of right kidney, between ascending and transverse colon, is covered by a layer of secondary parietal peritoneum derived from the ventral layer of the ascending mesocolon and continuous with the caudal layer of the transverse mesocolon. Beneath this secondary parietal peritoneum are two obliterated layers, on the one hand the dorsal layer of the mesocolon, on the other the visceral infra-colic duodenal serosa and the primitive prerenal parietal peritoneum.

In the further development of the adult human arrangement the changes below the level of the transverse colon and mesocolon result in the fixation of the ascending and descending colon to the background of the right and left lumbar regions. The opposed serous surfaces of the ascending and descending mesocola and of the dorsal parietal peritoneum adhere and the process also usually involves the dorsal visceral peritoneum of the ascending and descending colon, so that these portions of the gut obtain a fixed position.

Adhesion of the mesocolon to the dorsal body wall (parietal peritoneum) does not occur at all points at the same time. Usually adhesion proceeds from the midline laterad. The fixation of the ascending colon in the human embryo begins about the fourth month.

In the descending segment by the same time adhesion has usually proceeded nearly up to the descending colon, but the intestine itself is as yet free. In the fifth month the descending colon has usually become fixed between the splenic flexure and the beginning of the sigmoidea. In the latter region a free mesocolon usually persists throughout life.

Differences in the rate of growth between the length of the body wall and the length of the mesocolon may play an important part in the production of peritoneal *fossæ*, small pouches which in some regions of the abdomen may assume considerable proportions. Such fossæ are found around the duodeno-jejunal angle, the cæcum and appendix, and the sigmoid flexure. They will be considered more in detail with these respective regions, especially in reference to their relation to retro-peritoneal hernia.

In a certain proportion of cases adhesion between the parietal peritoneum and the ascending and descending mesocolon is incomplete or entirely wanting, resulting in the formation of a more or less completely free ascending and descending mesocolon. Treves, in an examination of 100 bodies, obtained the following figures:

In 52 subjects there was neither an ascending nor a descending mesocolon, the intestine being fixed in the manner which is regarded as normal.

In 22 there was a descending, but no trace of an ascending mesocolon.

In 14 a mesocolon was found in both the ascending and descending segments of the large intestine.

In 12 there was an ascending mesocolon, but no corresponding fold on the left side. Hence from this series a mesocolon may be expected on the left side in 36 per cent., on the right side in 26 per cent.

FIG. 155.—Abdominal viscera of *Macacus cynomolgus*, Kra monkey, hardened *in situ.* (Columbia University Museum, No. 1801.)

Both development and comparative anatomy would lead us to expect that the descending mesocolon would be found more frequently than the ascending.

In the lower animals the descending mesocolon is always an extensive and conspicuous membrane. It is well developed in all monkeys and the anthropoidea, as the remains of the primary vertical fold of the dorsal mesentery, while the ascending mesocolon is a secondary production, acquired during the development of the bowel by rotation.

In most of the lower monkeys the ascending mesocolon is also largely or entirely free. The descending mesocolon can always in these animals be reflected to the median line (cf. Fig. 155).

The line of attachment in man of the descending mesocolon is usually along the lateral border of the left kidney and vertical, while the line of attachment of the ascending mesocolon is usually less vertical, crossing the caudal end of the right kidney obliquely from right to left and with an upward direction (Fig. 156).

FIG. 156.—Schema of visceral and peritoneal relations of ventral surface of right kidney.

In like manner when both the ascending and descending mesocola are absent as free membranes the left or descending colon is adherent along the lateral border of the kidney to the abdominal parietes, while the ascending colon is fixed at the hepatic flexure a little obliquely across the ventral surface of the caudal end of the corresponding gland ascending toward the medial margin.

Treves found in the cases of persistent ascending mesocolon in the adult that the membrane varied in breadth from 1″ to 2″ while the persistent fold on the left side varied between 2″ and 3″ in breadth.

In the fœtus, up to 5″–6″ in length, the descending mesocolon is usually an extensive fold. Its attachment is vertical, but nearer to the median line than in the adult, usually along the medial border of the left kidney. It is at times found attached along this line in the adult.

An ascending mesocolon is rare even in the fœtus. The cæcum and beginning of the ascending colon are completely invested by peritoneum, but above the parts so invested the colon is usually adherent along an oblique line to the ventral and medial aspect of the right kidney.

In the fœtus at full term, if the cæcum is still undescended and in contact with the liver, it is not uncommon to find the cephalic portion of the descending colon provided with a mesocolon, while the caudal part of the descending colon is fixed by adhesion to the ventral surface and lateral border of the left kidney. This free membrane is then really a part of the transverse mesocolon. Where the cæcum descends to the iliac fossa the portion of the fœtal descending colon so invested is drawn over to the right and incorporated in the transverse colon.

Treves in two out of 100 bodies found the cæcum in the right iliac region, but both it and the whole of the ascending colon were entirely free from any peritoneal connections with the dorsal parietes of the abdomen.

The gut from the tip of the cæcum to the hepatic flexure was entirely invested by peritoneum continuous with the mesentery. The ascending colon was covered in the same manner and by the same fold as the small intestine. The segment of large intestine thus free measured 8″ in both instances.

The mesentery lacked the usual attachment to the dorsal abdominal wall and its root was represented by the interval between the duodenum and the transverse colon. The membrane had no other than its original primary attachment, and small intestine and ascending colon formed together a loop that practically represented the condition of the great primary intestinal loop. (Compare p. 73.)

The arrangement presented in these two subjects corresponds to that met in many animals, such as the cat.

A cross-section of the cat's abdomen arranged as above would show the following disposition of the peritoneum, corresponding to the stage in the human development preceding the fixation of the two vertical colic segments (Fig. 157). It will be seen that the right and left mesocola can be reflected to the median line where they become continuous ventrad of the vertebral column and aorta with the mesentery of the small intestine. The ventral surfaces of both kidneys are seen to be covered by the primitive parietal peritoneum of the abdominal cavity.

FIGS. 157, 158.—Schema showing peritoneal arrangement in transection of infra-colic compartment of abdomen before and after fixation of ascending and descending colon.

Fig. 158 shows the adult human arrangement of the same parts, after fixation of the vertical colic segments by adhesion of the opposed surfaces of their mesocola and the primitive parietal peritoneum. The background of the abdomen is now seen to be covered by a layer of secondary parietal peritoneum, *viz.*, the original left leaf of the ascending and right leaf of the descending mesocolon, continuous above with the lower or caudal layer of the transverse mesocolon.

This adhesion is so complete that the original condition is disregarded in adult descriptive anatomy. The layer which has adhered to the parietal peritoneum can no longer be recognized and the other has assumed the rôle of parietal peritoneum.

The connection of the transverse mesocolon with the dorsal lamella of the great omentum will be considered below.

The course of the vessels in the ascending and descending mesocola is not altered by the secondary adhesions. These vessels are in the adult situated behind the secondary parietal peritoneum derived from the mesocola.

The origin of the transverse mesocolon obtains by the fixation of the hepatic and splenic flexures high up in the abdomen a transverse course, and the transverse growth of the abdomen holds the membrane in this position cephalad of the duodeno-jejunal flexure, so that on elevating the transverse colon the mesocolon appears as separating the upper from the lower abdominal compartment. This posterior line of attachment or so-called "root of the transverse mesocolon," is nothing more than the upper limit of the area of adhesion between the primitive parietal peritoneum and the opposed surfaces of the ascending and descending mesocola. Reference to the abdominal cavity of the cat after complete rotation (Fig. 146) will show the original continuity of the three mesocola very clearly. A secondary connection is established along the lateral border of ascending and descending colon (Fig. 158), between the primitive parietal peritoneum and the ventral visceral peritoneal investment of the large intestine. Both of the vertical segments of the colon now appear fixed. Their dorsal surfaces are uncovered by peritoneum and can be reached in the lumbar region, laterad of the kidney, without opening the peritoneal cavity (lumbar colotomy).

The caudal portions of both kidneys are covered, beneath the secondary parietal peritoneum, by a layer of loose connective tissue representing the result of obliteration by adhesion of the first and second of the original three layers of prerenal peritoneum, viz., the primitive parietal (1) and the two layers of the mesocola (2 and 3).

LINE OF ATTACHMENT OF THE MESENTERY OF THE JEJUNO-ILEUM.—Examination of the caudal surface of the transverse mesocolon in the cat, with the parts in the above outlined position, will show how and why in the adult human abdomen the duodeno-jejunal angle appears to dip out from beneath the transverse mesocolon, becoming gradually more and more free until complete transition to the mobile jejunum is obtained. From this point, situated to the left of the second lumbar vertebra, the dorsal attachment of the adult human mesentery of the jejuno-ileum extends somewhat obliquely caudad and to the right to terminate in the right iliac fossa at the ileo-colic junction.

Returning to the conditions presented by the cat's intestines to obtain an explanation of this line of fixation we must recall the fact that in the peritoneum included within the limits of the umbilical loop, after differentiation of small and large intestine, but before rotation, we have both the elements of the mesentery of the small intestines and of the ascending and transverse mesocolon combined (Fig. 141). For it will be seen that this membrane carries at this time vessels both to the jejuno-ileum and to the segments of the large intestine (cæcum, ascending and transverse colon). This fact will be at once recognized if the cat's intestines are arranged to correspond to the primitive condition (Fig. 136) and the mesentery examined.

After rotation and differentiation of the colic segments and after the adhesion of the ascending and descending colon in man, the course of the main trunk of the superior mesenteric artery passes, after crossing the third portion of the duodenum, down and to the right to terminate near the ileo-colic junction by anastomosis with its ileo-colic branch. The adhesion of the right and left mesocola to the dorsal parietal peritoneum proceeds mesad as far as this line, leaving free the mesentery of the small intestines, which contains the vasa intestini tenuis derived from the left side of the main vessel. The secondary line of attachment of the mesentery to the abdominal background is therefore along this line. To obtain a clear idea of these processes of development in man assume that in the cat, after rotation and establishment of the three divisions of the colon, the two vertical (ascending and descending) mesocola become adherent to the dorsal parietal peritoneum, leaving the mesentery of the small intestine free.

FIG. 159.—Schematic figure to show lines of mesocolic adhesion, formation of root of transverse mesocolon and root of mesentery of jejuno-ileum in human subject.

Fig. 159 illustrates schematically the area of mesocolic adhesion in the human subject after complete rotation, and the line of the mesentery of jejuno-ileum.

Fixation of the ascending and descending cola and of their mesocola proceeds cephalad as far as the line AB, which thereby constitutes the root of the free transverse mesocolon.

The secondary parietal peritoneum derived from the ventral layer of the ascending mesocolon covers the lower and inner portion of the ventral surface of the right kidney, the infra-colic division of the descending and the dextro-mesenteric segment of the transverse duodenum, while along the root of the jejuno-ileal mesentery it becomes continuous with the right layer of that membrane. The secondary parietal peritoneum derived from the ventral layer of the descending colon covers the lower part of the ventral surface of the left kidney and the sinistro-mesenteric segment of the transverse duodenum and becomes continuous along the mesenteric radix with the left layer of the jejuno-ileal mesentery.

Caudad the adhesion of the descending colon and mesocolon to the parietal peritoneum proceeds only to the point C, following the dotted line mesad and resulting in the formation of the free mesocolon of the sigmoid flexure.

Résumé of the Adult Arrangement of the Human Peritoneum in the Lower Compartment of the Abdomen, Below the Level of the Transverse Colon and Mesocolon.—We should now consider the arrangement of the human peritoneum in the adult below the dorsal attachment of the transverse mesocolon in the light of the embryological and comparative anatomical facts just stated. In doing this it will be advisable to study both the actual conditions encountered and their significance in the sense of

40

determining the derivation of the peritoneal layers from the primitive dorsal mesentery. Open the abdominal cavity in the usual manner by a cruciform incision.

Turn the great omentum up on the chest wall, exposing the underlying intestines. This manipulation, as already stated, will cause the omentum to carry the transverse colon with it, on account of the adhesion, in the adult, of the gut to the dorsal layer of the omentum. Hence the cephalic or upper layer of the transverse mesocolon will not be seen at this stage because the omental adhesion just referred to prevents us from passing between the greater curvature of the stomach and the transverse colon without tearing peritoneal layers. It will, however, be possible to trace on the right side the duodenum from the pylorus down ventrad of the right kidney until the descending portion disappears behind the hepatic flexure of the colon. With the omentum and transverse mesocolon turned up, as stated, and the transverse mesocolon put upon the stretch, it will be seen that the abdominal space now overlooked is bounded cephalad by the lower layer of the transverse mesocolon and its attachment to the dorsal abdominal wall. The lateral limits of the space are given by the ascending and descending colon respectively. The attachment of the mesentery of the small intestine to the oblique line extending from the left of the vertebral column at about the level of the second lumbar vertebra to the right iliac fossa subdivides the entire space into a secondary right and left compartment.

Begin by following the caudal layer of the transverse mesocolon dorsad on the right side. In the angle between ascending and transverse colon (hepatic flexure) pressure will locate the caudal portion of the ventral surface of the right kidney. Remember that the peritoneum touched in these procedures appears in the adult as parietal prerenal peritoneum, but that in reality it is the left leaf of the originally free ascending mesocolon, whereas the original right leaf of this membrane and the primitive parietal peritoneum have, by adhesion of their serous surfaces, been converted into the loose subserous connective tissue covering the ventral aspect of the kidney beneath what now appears as parietal peritoneum.

Mesad of the resistance offered to the finger by the right kidney the caudal (infra-colic) portion of the descending duodenum and the angle of transition between it and the third or transverse portion will be found, invested in the same way by secondary (mesocolic) parietal peritoneum. It will be seen, especially if the duodenum is injected or inflated, that the hepatic flexure of the colon lies ventrad of the vertical descending second portion of the duodenum, so that one part of this intestine is situated cephalad the other caudad of the colon. (Supra- and infra-colic segments of descending duodenum.)

Individual differences are observed in the area of colic attachment to the duodenum. Usually the two intestines are in contact with each other and adherent over a considerable surface. Exceptionally the transverse mesocolon extends across to the right so as to include the hepatic flexure. In this latter case the uncovered non-peritoneal surface of the descending duodenum is small, represented by the interval between the layers of the transverse mesocolon, and the hepatic flexure is then not directly adherent to the gut.

If we now trace the transverse duodenum from right to left we will encounter the right layer of the root of the jejuno-ileal mesentery. The caudal layer of the transverse mesocolon, the right leaf of the mesentery and the secondary parietal peritoneum investing the ventral surface of the transverse duodenum all meet at this point. Surround the mesentery of the free small intestine with the fingers of one hand so that the entire mass of intestinal coils can be swung alternately from side to side.

Turning them over to the left, as already stated, the proximal portion of the transverse duodenum can be traced from right to left as far as the root of the mesentery. Here the peritoneum investing the ventral surface of the duodenum becomes continuous with the right leaf of the mesentery. Now swing the whole mass of small intestines over to the right, exposing the parietal peritoneum in the space to the left of the vertebral column, between the attachment of the mesentery to the median side, the root of transverse mesocolon cephalad and the descending colon to the left. Remember that the same significance attaches to this secondary parietal peritoneum as on the right side. It appears in the adult as parietal peritoneum, but is in its derivation the original right leaf of the descending mesocolon. Close to the root of the mesentery the continuation from the right side of the transverse duodenum will be seen, crossing the median line from right to left ventrad of aorta and vertebral column and usually turning cephalad on the left side of the lumbar vertebræ, as the fourth or ascending duodenum, to reach the caudal surface of the transverse mesocolon near its attachment, where the gut turns ventrad to form the duodeno-jejunal angle and become continuous with the free small intestine.

From the fact that the transverse duodenum is thus seen on each side of the root of the mesentery it will be recalled that after rotation of the primitive intestine the superior mesenteric artery crosses the transverse portion of the duodenum to reach its distribution between the leaves of the mesentery. Hence this portion of the small intestine consists of a dextro- and sinistro-mesenteric segment. This intersection of mesentery and duodenum marks the site of the primitive duodeno-colic isthmus through which the superior mesenteric artery passed to reach its distribution to the gut composing the embryonic umbilical loop.

To the left of the ascending duodenum a portion of the caudal surface of the pancreas will be seen, covered by the continuation of the caudal leaf of the transverse mesocolon into the parietal peritoneum. The consideration of this relation of peritoneum and pancreas will profitably be deferred until we have studied the developmental changes in the region of the dorsal mesogastrium and great omentum.

In the angle between termination of the transverse colon and proximal part of descending colon (splenic flexure) the caudal part of the ventral surface of the left kidney will be felt. The disposition of the peritoneum and its significance is the same as on the right side. Inasmuch as we have already seen that the secondary parietal peritoneum covering the dorsal abdominal wall on each side of the small intestine's mesenteric attachment is derived from the primitive ascending and descending mesocolon, it will be readily understood why the blood vessels supplying the ascending and descending colon (arteria ileo-colica, a. colica dextra, a. colica sinistra) are placed *behind* the parietal peritoneum, while the colica media, supplying the transverse colon, runs between the layers of the transverse mesocolon. Originally the same condition obtained for the two vertical colic segments, but with the anchoring of these portions of the large intestine and the adhesion of their mesocola to the parietal peritoneum the blood vessels which formerly ran between the two layers of the membrane, as long as it remained free, now appear as retroperitoneal vessels placed beneath the parietal peritoneum derived secondarily from the mesocola.

This fact must be borne in mind in studying the arrangement of certain folds and fossæ of the parietal peritoneum which are now to be considered.

Duodenal Fossæ. Fossa of Treitz and Retro-peritoneal Hernia.—The peritoneal cavity of the cat can be used to great advantage in order to obtain a clear idea of the formation of these folds and fossæ, whose relation to the so-called "retro-peritoneal hernia" has led to an exaggerated elaboration of minute detail and a somewhat puzzling terminology in human descriptive anatomy.

FIG. 160.—Abdominal cavity of cat, with intestines everted and elevated to show duodenal fold. (From a fresh dissection.)

FIG. 161.—Abdominal viscera of *Nasua rufa*, brown coaiti. (From a fresh dissection.)

FIG. 162.—Abdominal viscera of *Hapale vulgaris*, the marmoset. (Columbia University Museum, No. 1818.)

FIG. 163.—Abdominal viscera of cat; intestines rotated and turned to the right to show duodenal fold. (From a fresh dissection.)

Directions for Examining the Folds and the Formation of the Duodeno-jejunal Fossa in the Cat.—Turn the omentum and the coils of the small intestine cephalad out of the abdomen until they rest upon the ventral thoracic wall. Press the large intestine over to the left side, putting the mesocolon on the stretch until the parts are arranged as shown in Fig. 160. The loop of the duodenum with the head portion of the pancreas will be seen caudad of the liver and ventrad of the right kidney. A well-marked peritoneal fold, somewhat sickle-shaped, with the concavity of the free edge directed caudad and to the right, will be seen extending from the convex border of the duodenum, directly opposite the mesenteric or attached margin, to the right leaf of the mesocolon. This fold indicates the beginning adhesion of the duodenum to the mesocolic peritoneum, the first step toward the subsequent complete fixation of the gut as it is found in man.

Fig. 161 shows the abdominal cavity of Nasua rufa, the brown Coati-mundi, a South American arctoid carnivore, with the intestines everted and turned to the left side. In this animal the large intestine is very short, there is no cæcum, the ileo-colic junction is only marked on the surface by a pyloric-like constriction of the tube and in the interior by the projection of a ring-valve (Fig. 408).

The duodenal fold is very well developed, passing between the convex surface of the duodenal loop and the adjacent right leaf of the short mesocolon.

In Primates, in which complete rotation of the intestine, on the plan of the human development, takes place, still further and more extensive agglutination of the serous surface of the duodenum to the peritoneum of the mesocolon occurs. Fig. 162 shows the condition in *Hapale vulgaris*, one of the marmosets. The ascending and descending mesocola and the mesoduodenum of this animal are still free, but the surface of the duodenum has become fastened to the opposed mesocolon. With fixation of the hepatic flexure and adhesion of the ascending colon, such as occurs in man, the duodenum is carried dorsad against the ventral surface of the right kidney, and now anchoring of the duodenum, by obliteration of the mesoduodenum and adhesion to the prerenal parietal peritoneum, takes place as already detailed above. To return now to the formation of the duodeno-jejunal fossa by means of this fold, as illustrated in the cat. Perform the manipulations already described in rotation of the intestine. The appearance of the parts then will be as shown in Fig. 163. The large intestine is drawn over so as to represent the human ascending and transverse colon in one segment, the descending colon in the other, and the mesocolon appears correspondingly as transverse and descending. In other words the cat's intestines as arranged in the figure would represent the stage in the human development in which cæcum and beginning of large intestine are still subhepatic in position ventrad of the right kidney, before differentiation of ascending and transverse colon by descent of cæcum into right iliac fossa.

In the human subject, as we have seen, the transverse mesocolon obtains a secondary attachment to the background of the abdominal cavity, its caudal surface remaining free.

The descending mesocolon turns its original right leaf ventrad, its left leaf dorsad, and the latter adheres to the primitive parietal peritoneum covering the left lumbar region and ventral surface of left kidney. This area of adhesion extends up to and usually involves the dorsal surface of the descending colon, anchoring the same in the left lumbar region, down to the point where the sigmoid flexure begins and where the original mesocolon again appears free.

In the cat, therefore, with the intestines arranged to correspond to the course of the human large intestine after rotation has been accomplished, the lines representing the peritoneal human adhesions should be fixed, as shown in the schema, Fig. 159: AB, line of secondary attachment after rotation resulting in the formation of the "root" of a free transverse mesocolon. BC, line of limit of secondary adhesion to the original parietal peritoneum involving the entire left (now dorsal) layer of the descending mesocolon and the dorsal surface of the descending colon, resulting in the fixation of the latter part of the large intestine.

This establishes, as already stated, a secondary parietal peritoneal surface in the left lumbar region derived from the original right leaf of the descending mesocolon. Inasmuch as the inferior mesenteric vessels originally passed to the descending colon between the layers of the mesocolon they will now apparently be placed beneath the (secondary) parietal peritoneum of the left lumbar region.

If now the duodenal fold in the cat be examined after rotation of the intestine it will be found presenting the original relations (Figs. 160 and 163), viz., passing from the convex margin of that portion of the duodenal loop which would correspond to the human fourth or ascending portion, to the original right layer of the mesocolon, which in man becomes secondarily converted into the parietal peritoneum of the left lumbar region. Hence the connections of the fold are as follows:

On the right: ventral surface of the ascending duodenum.

On the left: right layer of mesocolon (secondary lumbar parietal peritoneum in the adult human subject).

Cephalad it abuts against the caudal layer of the transverse mesocolon along the line which would correspond to the root of the mesocolon in the adult human subject.

The concave *caudal* edge is free and bounds the entrance into a fossa, the "superior duodenal fossa" of anthropotomy. This fossa opens caudad and extends cephalad to the root of the transverse mesocolon. The ventral and left wall of the fossa is formed by the fold in question, its background by the mesocolon (right leaf); to the right the left circumference of the ascending duodenum enters into the formation of the fossa, and its fundus is formed by the confluence of the fold and of the caudal layer of the transverse mesocolon. The inferior mesenteric vessels are found near the left margin of the entrance into the fossa.

FIG. 164.—Abdominal viscera of *Nasua rufa*, the brown coaiti, showing the position of the duodenal fold after rotation of the intestine. (From a fresh dissection.)

FIG. 165.—Abdominal viscera of human fœtus at term, arranged to show duodenal folds and fossa. The jejuno-ileum, ascending and transverse colon have been removed. (Columbia University Museum, No. 1819.)

Fig. 164 shows the appearance of the fold in *Nasua rufa* after rotation of the intestine. The short course of the large intestine in this animal, and the consequent reduction of the mesocolon, brings the fold much below the level which it occupies in the cat.

If we now look for the corresponding structures in man we will find certain modifications depending chiefly upon still closer adhesion between duodenum and the mesocolon which is destined to become the left parietal peritoneum after anchoring of the descending colon. We have already encountered an example of such closer connection in the marmoset shown in Fig. 162.

In all cases the "superior duodenal" fold, corresponding to the fold just encountered in the cat, is the original condition, and the duodenal fossa consequently opens caudad. In many instances this will be the only fold and fossa encountered in the adult human subject. In other instances more extensive duodeno-mesocolic adhesions result in the addition of an "inferior fold," bounding a fossa the entrance into which is directed cephalad toward the transverse mesocolon. Such a condition is seen in Fig. 165 taken from a fœtus at term. The duodenal fossa in this case is bounded by an "upper" and "lower" duodenal fold continuous with each other on the left side, but separated on the right at their attachment to the duodenum. It will be seen that the inferior mesenteric vein runs in the left margin of the fold, following along the left border of the entrance into the fossa. A segment of the colica sinistra artery may occupy the same position. This position of the vein, or artery, or of both vessels, is not the cause leading to the formation of the duodenal fossa, but is more or less accidental and variable. In many cases the vessels run at some distance from the folds bounding the fossa.

In some subjects the "inferior" fold is the only one found, and the only duodenal fossa then encountered looks cephalad. This condition, when associated with the course of the inferior mesenteric vessels in the free edge of the fold, constituted the classical "fossa duodeno-jejunalis" of Treitz, and is described as "Treitz's fossa."

FIG. 166.—Abdominal viscera of human fœtus at term. (Columbia University Museum, No. 1820.)

FIG. 167.—Abdominal viscera of adult human subject, showing duodenal folds and fossa. (From a fresh dissection.)

FIG. 168.—Abdominal viscera of adult human subject, showing duodenal folds and fossa. (From a fresh dissection.)

Fig. 166 shows the condition in which only a small inferior fold attaches itself to the termination of the transverse duodenum. There is practically an entire absence of duodenal or duodeno-jejunal folds and fossæ. The inferior mesenteric vessels course under cover of the mesocolic secondary parietal peritoneum, but do not produce a fold.

Fig. 167, from an adult human subject, illustrates the further development of the fossa from the fœtal conditions shown in Fig. 165. The well-marked duodenal fossa is bounded by a superior and inferior duodenal fold, uniting laterally in a crescentic margin containing a segment of the inferior mesenteric vein and colica sinistra artery. The lower division of the peritoneal recess thus produced corresponds to the typical (vascular) "fossa of Treitz." Mesally the projection of the fourth portion of the duodenum bounds the fossa.

In Fig. 168, also taken from an adult human subject, an extensive duodenal recess is bounded in the same way by a superior and inferior duodenal fold. In the interior of the fossa a third duodenal reduplication of the peritoneum ("intermediate duodenal fold") is seen, as is also the trunk of the inferior mesenteric vein, while the main trunk of the colica sinistra artery courses laterally behind the secondary mesocolic parietal peritoneum near the margin of the descending colon.

It will be seen that the freedom of the ascending or fourth portion of the duodenum depends largely upon the disposition and extent of these folds. Inasmuch as they are the product of varying degrees of adhesion of this segment of the intestine they are subject to great individual variations and have given rise to an unnecessary and complicated classification of the duodenal folds and fossæ. The close relation maintained between the duodeno-jejunal angle and the caudal layer of the transverse mesocolon near its root at times leads to the production of a peritoneal fold connecting this membrane with the duodeno-jejunal knuckle of intestine (duodeno-jejunal or mesocolic fold) and may result in the formation of a duodeno-jejunal or mesocolic fossa of the peritoneum. An instance of this fold is seen inFig. 168.

The importance of the duodenal fossæ, and of similar peritoneal recesses in other parts of the abdominal cavity, is founded on the fact that by gradual enlargement they may lodge the greater part of the movable small intestine in their interior, leading to the formation of intra- or retro-peritoneal herniæ.[3]

Fossa Intersigmoidea.—A second peritoneal pocket or fossa is encountered in the region of the sigmoid flexure and its mesocolon. The formation of this fossa is closely associated with the adult disposition of the sigmoid mesocolon as part of the original primitive vertical dorsal mesentery. In the typical arrangement of the parts the sigmoid or omega loop of the large intestine has a free mesocolon. The adhesion of the descending mesocolon to the parietal peritoneum usually ceases along a line drawn horizontally from the lateral margin of the left psoas at a level with the crest of the ilium to the medial side of the iliac vessels. This line, along which the mesocolon ceases to be adherent to the parietal peritoneum, joins the attachment of the distal portion of the sigmoid mesocolon, which partially retains its primitive vertical origin to the dorsal midline, at a right angle. This angle is the site of the*intersigmoid fossa*, the entrance into which is seen usually as a round opening of variable size on elevating the sigmoid flexure and putting its mesocolon on the stretch. Fig. 159shows the area of adhesion between the primitive descending mesocolon and the parietal peritoneum (from C mesad) which results in the formation of a free mesocolon for the sigmoid flexure. Frequently in the angle formed by the horizontal and vertical line of attachment of the sigmoid mesocolon a non-adherent strip of the primitive mesocolon roofs in a more or less extensive intersigmoid fossa, whose fundus is directed upwards and inwards.

Cæcum, Appendix and Ileo-colic Junction.—Several peritoneal fossæ and folds are found in the ileo-colic region in connection with the cæcum, appendix and termination of the ileum. The practical importance of this portion of the intestinal tract and the great morphological interest which attaches to the same make it worth while to consider its anatomy in a separate chapter.

PART II.

ANATOMY OF THE PERITONEUM IN THE SUPRA-COLIC
COMPARTMENT OF THE ABDOMEN.

We have already seen that the transverse colon and mesocolon effect a general division of the adult human abdominal cavity into a cephalic supra-colic compartment, situated between the diaphragm and the level of the transverse colon and mesocolon, comprising in general the hypochondriac and epigastric regions, and a larger caudal infra-colic space which includes the entire rest of the abdominal cavity and is continued caudad into the pelvic cavity. The arrangement of the peritoneum and viscera in this latter space has just been considered. The fact will be recalled that the second or descending portion of the duodenum, passing dorsad of the hepatic colic flexure, forms so to speak the visceral connection between the portions of the alimentary tube situated in the supra-colic compartment and those situated in the infra-colic space. The fixation of this segment of the duodenum and its consequent secondary retroperitoneal position in the adult human subject masks this continuity of the alimentary canal to a certain extent so that it requires more than a superficial examination in order to trace correctly the course of the duodenum from the pylorus to the duodeno-jejunal angle, dorsad of the colon, root of transverse mesocolon and mesentery, and under cover of the secondary parietal peritoneum.

We have now to turn our attention to the viscera contained in the cephalic or supra-colic compartment of the abdomen and to consider the disposition of the serous membrane investing them and connecting them with each other and with the abdominal parietes.

The visceral contents of the supra-colic compartment comprise the liver, pancreas, spleen, stomach and the proximal portion of the duodenum, including the hepatic angle and the supra-colic part of the descending duodenum. Less directly the cephalic portions of the right and left kidney and the corresponding suprarenal capsules belong to this visceral group.

In this region of the abdomen we meet with the most extensive modifications of the primitive dorsal peritoneal membrane, producing conditions which, considered without reference to development and comparative anatomy, are complex and difficult of comprehension. These changes lead to the formation of the so-called "lesser sac," a term which in some respects is unfortunate as it implies a more complete degree of separation from the general peritoneal cavity or "greater sac" than actually exists.

In order to clearly understand the adult arrangement of the peritoneum in this region it is advisable to consider the subject in two distinct subdivisions, dealing successively with the two cardinal facts which contribute to effect the change from the simple primitive to the complicated adult condition.

These two main elements are:

1. Developmental changes in the position of the stomach, alterations in the disposition of the proximal part of the primitive dorsal mesentery attached to the stomach, and the development of pancreas and spleen in connection with this membrane.

2. The development of the liver and the successive stages in the production of the final adult vascular and serous relations of this organ.

1. Stomach and Dorsal Mesogastrium.—We have already considered the early stages in the differentiation of the stomach from the primitive intestinal tube of uniform caliber (p. 40). It will be recalled that the stomach at a certain period, while it already presents the main structural features familiar in the adult organ, occupies a vertical position in the abdominal cavity, turning its concave margin (lesser curvature) ventrad, while the convex dorsal border (greater curvature) is directed toward the vertebral column, being attached to the same by the layers of the proximal part of the primitive dorsal mesentery. At this time the stomach presents right and left surfaces, and the œsophageal entrance is at the highest or cephalic point of the organ, while the pyloric transition to the small intestine occupies the distal caudal extremity.

The primitive dorsal mesentery, as already stated, passes as a thin double-layered membrane between the ventral surface of the vertebral column and the dorsal border of the stomach, which, as we will presently see, becomes during the later stages of development the caudal (lower) margin or greater curvature.

It will be seen that the embryonic differentiation of the intestinal tract into successive segments justifies the application of a terminology based on this differentiation to the corresponding portions of the primitive common dorsal mesentery.

Thus the proximal portion extending between the vertebral column and the dorsal border or greater curvature of the stomach becomes the *mesogastrium*; we differentiate this portion still further as the *"dorsal mesogastrium"* to distinguish it from a *"ventral mesogastrium"* which we will presently encounter in considering the development of the liver and the connected peritoneum.

In the same way the section of the primitive common dorsal mesentery attached to the duodenal loop becomes the *mesoduodenum*, that connected with the mobile part of the small intestine (jejuno-ileum) the *mesentery* proper, while the portion passing to the colon forms the *mesocolon*, to be subsequently still further subdivided, after the different segments of the large intestine have become mapped out, as the *ascending, transverse* and *descending mesocolon*, the *mesosigmoidea* and the *mesorectum.*

In tracing the development of the adult human peritoneum it is well to consider certain stages, which we will find illustrated by the permanent conditions presented by some of the lower vertebrates:

These stages comprise:

(*a*) Changes in the position of the stomach.

(*b*) Changes in the direction and extent of the dorsal mesogastrium.

(*c*) Development of the pancreas and spleen in connection with the mesogastrium.

A. Changes in the Position of the Stomach.

The primitive position of the organ above outlined (p. 41) is changed during the course of further development by a twofold rotation.

1. The primitive vertical position, in which the œsophageal entrance occupies the highest cephalic extremity, while the pyloric opening is at the opposite caudal end, is exchanged for one directed more transversely, approximating the two gastric orifices to the same horizontal level. In human embryos of 13.9 mm. the fundus has already descended, the pylorus moving cephalad and to the right, while the cardia becomes shifted more to the left. At the same time the greater growth and prominence of the convex border or greater curvature becomes marked in comparison with the relatively short extent of the opposite margin or lesser curvature.

FIGS. 169, 170.—Two front views of the entodermal canal. (Minot, after His.)

FIG. 169.—Embryo Sch. 1 of   FIG. 170.—Embryo Sch. 2 of His.   His.

2. Coincident with this change in position is a rotation around the vertical axis, by means of which the original left side of the stomach is turned ventrad, becoming the ventral or "anterior" surface, while the original right surface of the organ now looks dorsad toward the vertebral column, becoming the dorsal or "posterior" surface of human anatomy. The œsophageal or cephalic end is placed to the left of the median line, while the caudal or pyloric end is situated on the right side (Figs. 169 and 170).

The original ventral border, now the "lesser curvature" or "upper border," looks cephalad and to the right, toward the caudal surface of the liver, while the original dorsal border, as the "greater curvature" or "lower border" is directed in the main caudad and to the left.

The prominence of this border is still further increased by the greater development of the stomach to the left of the œsophageal entrance resulting in the formation of the "fundus" or "great cul-de-sac."

This rotation of the stomach explains the asymmetrical position of the vagus nerve in the adult, the left side of the embryonic stomach, innervated by the left vagus, becoming the "anterior" surface of adult descriptive anatomy and *vice versa.*

It will be readily appreciated that a comparatively flat organ like the stomach, will, as long as it occupies a sagittal position, with right and left surfaces, help to divide the upper part of the abdominal cavity to a certain extent into a right and left half, even if the peritoneal connections of the organ are left out of consideration. As soon, however, as the above-described changes in position take place and the surfaces of the stomach are directed ventrad and dorsad, the relative arrangement and extent of this right and left abdominal space becomes altered by the different disposition of the septum, *i. e.*, the stomach. The original right side of the organ is now directed dorsad, and the rotation of the organ has created a space between this dorsal or "posterior" surface of the stomach and the background of the abdominal cavity, which is the inception of the "lesser peritoneal cavity" or retrogastric space. We will find that this space becomes well defined and circumscribed by the peritoneal connections of the stomach, but we will realize, even at this stage, that the *dorsal* surface of the stomach will form a part of the general *ventral* wall of the lesser peritoneal space.

47

On the other hand, the partial division of the abdomen into a right and left half, effected by the stomach in its primitive sagittal position, disappears after rotation of the organ. We now pass uninterruptedly from left to right across the ventral (original *left*) surface of the stomach.

B. Changes in the Direction and Extent of the Dorsal Mesogastrium.

The effects of the altered position of the stomach on the disposition of the abdominal space have just been considered in relation to the organ itself, without reference to its natural connections with the parietes and with adjacent viscera. Their true significance and their influence on the adult anatomical arrangement of the abdomen is, however, only appreciated when the changes in the arrangement of the peritoneal membrane which they involve, are taken into account.

The dorsal mesogastrium changes more than any other portion of the peritoneum in the course of development. It not only becomes displaced and altered in direction by the rotation of the stomach, but in addition it grows so extensively that it finally hangs down like an apron over the entire mass of small intestines, forming the great omentum.

FIG. 171.—Schematic   FIG. 172.—Semi-diagrammatic representation of dorsal mesogastrium representation of mesogastrium in human embryo before rotation of stomach. of the sixth week. (Kollmann.)

If we begin with the primitive disposition of the sagittal stomach and dorsal mesogastrium shown in Fig. 171 it will be observed that both structures together actually divide the dorsal portion of the abdominal cavity into symmetrical right and left halves (Fig. 172).

After rotation of the stomach (Fig. 173) the mesogastrium loses its original sagittal direction. It follows the altered position of the original dorsal border of the stomach, which has now become the caudal margin or "greater curvature," by turning caudad and to the left, being at the same time considerably elongated. This occurs during the second month. Hence the dorsal mesogastrium, after leaving the vertebral column, turns ventrad and to the left to reach its gastric attachment along the greater curvature. This is the first indication of the formation of the great omental or epiploic bursa.

FIGS. 173-175.—Schema of dorsal mesogastrium after rotation of stomach.

FIG. 173.—Early stage.

FIG. 174.—Later stage, extension of mesogastrium beyond stomach to left, with fundus of blind retrogastric pouch thus created at X.

FIG. 175.—After adhesion over area of dotted line between dorsal mesogastrium and primitive parietal peritoneum. Secondary line of transition from dorsal mesogastrium to parietal peritoneum at X.

FIG. 176.—Schematic ventral view of stomach, duodenum, and dorsal mesogastrium, after rotation of stomach and extension of omental bursa caudad beyond greater curvature of stomach. The ventral mesogastrium is detached along the lesser curvature.

FIG. 177.—Semi-diagrammatic representation of peritoneal membrane in human embryo. (After Kollmann.)

The stomach is here considered as developing in situ and as influencing by its growth and change of position the arrangement and direction of the peritoneal layers with which it is connected. As a matter of fact it is well to note that the stomach at first lies above the primitive diaphragm or septum transversum, migrating, however, at an early period into the subhepatic abdominal position. This migration produces a corresponding increase in the length of the œsophagus (Fig. 34) and the stomach, in consequence of this change in position, acquires its ventral and dorsal mesogastrium. For the purpose of explaining the adult peritoneal relations of the organ it is, however, more convenient to regard the stomach as an abdominal organ from the beginning and to deal with the subsequent changes in position from this standpoint. The inaccuracy is slight and renders the comprehension of the succeeding stages easier.

48

It will be noticed (Fig. 173) that the rudimentary retro-gastric space or "lesser peritoneal sac" is bounded ventrally by the dorsal (the primitive *right*) surface of the stomach, while its dorsal boundary is furnished by the ventral (originally *right*) layer of the dorsal mesogastrium.

In the primitive condition, therefore, dorsal mesogastrium and stomach form together a straight line sagittal in direction and placed in the median plane of the body. As the result of the developmental changes above outlined this straight line becomes bent at the point where the mesogastrium reaches the stomach (Fig. 173, x). The two component elements of the line (stomach and mesogastrium) hinge on each other here, and the angle which they form opens to the right.

The changes which are to be observed in the later stages depend principally upon a peculiar feature characteristic of the development of the dorsal mesogastrium. This feature consists in the extreme redundancy of the membrane which grows out of proportion to the requirements of its visceral connections, and to a certain extent becomes independent of the direct mechanical purpose of carrying blood vessels to the viscera. Hence in a transverse section at this period (Figs. 174 and 175) the mesogastrium no longer passes in a direct line between its points of attachment, viz. the greater curvature of the stomach and the vertebral column, but extends beyond the stomach to the left. We will appreciate the significance of this extensive growth of the mesogastrium especially in considering the development of the spleen and pancreas. For the present it will suffice to note (Figs. 174 and 175) that the growth has carried the mesogastrium well to the left of the stomach, consequently the retrogastric space is now bounded toward the left by the bend which the original right leaf of the primitive sagittal mesogastrium takes in order to reach its gastric attachment. The retrogastric space therefore terminates toward the left in a blind pocket formed by this reduplication of the mesogastrium.

One more factor is to be taken into consideration, namely the tendency, already noted, of peritoneal surfaces to become adherent to each other. Such adhesion involves the apposed surfaces of the mesogastrium and of the primitive parietal peritoneum to the left of the vertebral column. The dorsal (original *left*) layer of the mesogastrium adheres to the parietal peritoneum covering the left side of the abdominal background and the cephalic portion of the ventral surface of the left kidney up to the end of the blind pouch which forms the extreme left limit of the retrogastric space. Hence, after this process of adhesion is completed, the dorsal wall of the retrogastric space is lined by secondary parietal peritoneum covering the left kidney (original right leaf of primitive mesogastrium) (Fig. 175). We obtain (Fig. 175 at x) an apparent continuity of the parietal peritoneum with that portion of the mesogastrium which, derived from the original left layer of the membrane, appears now to extend, as the ventral one of two layers, between the stomach and the abdominal parietes near the lateral border of the left kidney. (Primitive gastro-splenic omentum.)

It should be remembered that the disposition of the peritoneum just indicated is modified by the development of the pancreas and spleen, both of which organs are intimately associated with the mesogastrium. The foregoing statements and diagrams are therefore merely given for the purpose of affording a general view of the extent, growth and changes of the dorsal mesogastrium before proceeding to consider the development of the pancreas and spleen in and from the membrane itself.

In the view directly from in front the redundancy of the peritoneum forming the mesogastrium is shown in Figs. 176 and 177. Just as the membrane extends further to the left than required by its visceral connection with the stomach, so the downward growthexceeds the demand made by the rotation of the attached border (greater curvature) caudad and to the left. The mesogastrium, forming, as it now does, the great omentum, enlarges in descending toward the transverse colon (Fig. 177). The bag thus formed can be distended with air in a fœtus of from 8 to 9 cm. vertex-coccygeal measure, as shown in the figure. Consequently in sagittal section the membrane is seen to extend caudad beyond the level of the greater curvature, and must turn on itself and pass again cephalad in order to reach the stomach (Fig. 178). By reason of this excessive growth the limits of the primitive retrogastric space are enlarged, not only toward the left, but more especially in the caudal direction. The bend made by the mesogastrium in returning to the stomach forms the blind

49

extremity of a pouch which continues the retrogastric space caudad beyond the stomach, and whose dorsal and ventral walls are formed by the reduplicated mesogastrium. This pocket or pouch constitutes the *omental* or *epiploic bursa* of the lesser peritoneal cavity, for the great omentum is the direct product of this redundant growth of the mesogastrium caudad. It will be observed that the great omentum is made up of four peritoneal layers, the folding of the double-layered mesogastrium naturally producing this result. The first or ventral and the fourth or dorsal layer are derived from the original left layer of the primitive sagittal mesogastrium; the intermediate second and third layers, separated from each other at this stage by the cavity of the omental bursa, are products of the primitive right leaf of the mesogastrium. Since the entire retrogastric space with its extensions becomes the "lesser cavity" of the human adult peritoneum, it will be seen that its serous membrane is derived from the original right leaf of the mesogastrium (second and third omental layers). After the above-described adhesion of the mesogastrium to the parietal peritoneum overlying the ventral surface of the left kidney, the membrane would be traced in sagittal section (Fig. 179) from the dorsal surface of the stomach caudad, lining the interior of the omental bursa (second layer) to the turn or blind end of the pouch; thence cephalad as the third omental layer, forming the dorsal wall of the epiploic bursa, to invest, as secondary parietal peritoneum, the cephalic segment of the ventral surface of the left kidney.

FIG. 178.—Schematic sagittal section through stomach and dorsal mesogastrium, after rotation and formation of omental bursa.

FIG. 179.—Schematic sagittal section through stomach and dorsal mesogastrium after adhesion to prerenal parietal peritoneum.

C. Development of Spleen and Pancreas in the Dorsal Mesogastrium and Changes in the Disposition of the Great Omentum.

In order to obtain a correct conception of the adult human conditions it is finally necessary to consider the development of the spleen and pancreas in their connection with the dorsal mesogastrium and to note the changes which are produced by adhesion of portions of the great omentum to adjacent serous surfaces. It will be advisable to discuss these subjects at first separately, and to subsequently combine all the facts in an attempt to gain a correct impression of their share in determining the disposition of the adult human peritoneum.

1. Development of Spleen.—The spleen develops from the mesoderm between the layers of the dorsal mesogastrium, near its point of accession to the greater curvature, in the region of the subsequent fundus. It has therefore, like the stomach, originally free peritoneal surfaces. After rotation of the stomach the organ lies between the two layers of the membrane at the extreme left end of the retrogastric space (Fig. 180).

FIG. 180.—Schematic transverse section of the abdomen, showing early stage of development of spleen from extreme left end of dorsal mesogastric pouch.

Vascular Connections.—The splenic artery accedes to the mesal surface of the spleen from the vessel which originally passed directly to the dorsal border (subsequent greater curvature) of the stomach, between the layers of the mesogastrium.

With the further growth of the spleen the segment of this vessel situated between its origin from the cœliac axis and the hilum of the spleen becomes relatively larger, forming the adult splenic artery, while the continuation of the original vessel to the greater curvature of the stomach appears now as a branch of the splenic artery, viz., the arteria gastro-epiploica sinistra.

Through the development of the spleen the dorsal mesogastrium has been subdivided into a proximal longer vertebro-splenic, and a distal shorter gastro-splenic segment. The former, as we have seen, loses its identity as a free membrane in the human adult, by fusing with the parietal peritoneum investing the ventral surface of the left kidney. Hence, after this adhesion has taken place, the splenic artery courses from the cœliac axis to the spleen behind peritoneum which functions as part of the general parietal membrane, but which is derived from the original right leaf of the proximal vertebro-splenic segment of the primitive mesogastrium (Fig. 181). On the other hand the distal segment of this membrane, beyond

50

the spleen, remains free, carrying, as the gastro-splenic omentum, the left gastro-epiploic artery between its layers from the splenic artery to the greater curvature of the stomach.

FIG. 181.—Schematic transverse section of the abdomen, showing later stage of development of spleen and arrangement of peritoneum after adhesion of dorsal layer of mesogastrium and primitive prerenal parietal peritoneum.

The lateral limit of the area of adhesion between mesogastrium and parietal peritoneum is situated along the lateral border of the left kidney. Hence, in the final condition of the parts, the main splenic vessels at the hilum are situated between two peritoneal layers of which the ventral (Fig. 181) appears as the parietal peritoneum forming the dorsal wall of the retro-gastric space, while the dorsal layer (Fig. 181) forms a reflection from the mesal surface of the spleen, along the dorsal margin of the hilum, to the adjacent lateral border of the left kidney (lieno-renal ligament) and to the diaphragm. At this point of adhesion subsequently firmer strands of connective tissue develop in the serous reduplication forming the *ligamentum phrenico-lienale* of systematic anatomy. This process of adhesion takes place during the second half of intra-uterine life. A connection with the colon, produced by adhesion of the mesogastrium to the splenic flexure of the large intestine, forms the adult *lig. colico-lienale*, while a similar adhesion between great omentum, transverse mesocolon and phrenic parietal peritoneum just caudad of the spleen, gives rise to the *colico-phrenic* or *costo-colic "supporting" ligament* of the spleen.

FIG. 182.—Part of the abdominal viscera of child, two years old, hardened *in situ* and removed from body. The great omentum has been detached along the line of the transverse colon. (Columbia University, Study Collection.)

FIG. 183.—The same preparation with the spleen removed, showing lines of peritoneal reflection on mesial surface of the organ.

On the other hand, the ventral one of the two layers constituting the gastro-splenic omentum and including between them the left gastro-epiploic artery, is formed by the distal part of the primitive left layer of the mesogastrium, while the dorsal layer of the same fold is the portion of the primitive right layer beyond the spleen, which has not been converted into secondary parietal peritoneum, but forms now part of the ventral wall of the lesser peritoneal sac between the spleen and the stomach (Fig. 181) (lig. gastro-lienale). Since, therefore, the gastro-splenic omentum is a specialized part of the fully-developed dorsal mesogastrium, and since we have seen that the great omentum is formed directly by the excessive growth of this membrane caudad, it is not difficult to understand why in the adult human subject the ventral layer of the gastro-splenic omentum is directly continuous with the ventral layer of the great omentum along the greater curvature of the stomach to which both are attached. The dorsal layer of the gastro-splenic omentum would, in the same way, be continuous with the second layer of the great omentum, lining the ventral wall of the omental bursa, if it were not for the fact that in the adult adhesions usually obliterate the cavity of the bursa.

Fig. 182 shows the stomach, left kidney, spleen and splenic flexure of the colon hardened in situ and removed from the body of a two-year-old child. The great omentum has been divided along the line of adherence to the transverse colon.

In Fig. 183 the spleen has been removed from the preparation by division of its peritoneal and vascular connections, and is shown in its mesal aspect (gastric and renal surfaces, intermediate margin and hilum). It will be seen that the peritoneal reflections are arranged in the form of two concentric elliptical lines. The two ventral lines form the gastro-splenic omentum and correspond to the reflection of the peritoneum from spleen to left end of stomach carrying the gastric branches derived from the splenic artery. The third line from before backwards results from the division of the secondary parietal peritoneum of the lesser sac, covering splenic artery, and ventral surface of pancreas and derived from the dorsal mesogastrium; while the most dorsal fourth line represents the divided reflection of the peritoneum from the renal surface of spleen to lateral border of left kidney and diaphragm (lig. lieno-renale).

Between the second and third lines of peritoneal reflection appears the portion of the mesal surface of the spleen in contact with and invested by the extreme left end of the lesser peritoneal sac.

Fig. 184, taken from an adult human subject with the viscera hardened in situ, shows the left or splenic extension of the lesser peritoneal cavity.

FIG. 184.—Upper abdominal viscera of adult human subject, hardened *in situ*, with liver and colon removed and stomach turned up. (Columbia University, Study Collection.)

FIG. 185.—Pancreatic and hepatic buds of human embryo of four weeks. (Kollmann.)

2. Development of the Pancreas.—The pancreatic gland is derived from the hypoblast of the enteric tube. The secreting epithelium and that lining the ducts of the adult gland is formed by budding and proliferation of the intestinal epithelium. The gland develops primarily from two outgrowths which are at first separate and distinct from each other.

1. The proximal and dorsal bud grows directly from the hypoblast lining the duodenum immediately beyond the pyloric junction.

In embryos of 8 mm. (four weeks) (Fig. 185) it appears as a small spherical outgrowth connected by a slightly narrower stalk with the epithelial intestinal tube.

2. The distal and ventral outgrowth is separated from the preceding and is from the beginning closely connected with the similar embryonic outgrowth from the enteric tube which is to form the liver. This portion of the pancreas is, strictly speaking, derived primarily from the epithelium of the primitive hepatic duct and not directly from the duodenum. This primary arrangement of the gland, being formed of two main collections of budding hypoblastic cells, corresponds to the adult system of the pancreatic excretory ducts. The proximal or dorsal outgrowth furnishes that portion of the head of the gland whose excretory system terminates in the *secondary pancreatic duct* or *duct of Santorini*, while the distal (ventral) outgrowth includes within its area the termination of the principal pancreatic duct or *canal of Wirsung*, which is closely connected with the end of the common bile-duct at the intestinal opening common to both (Figs. 186-187). The method of union of the two pancreatic outgrowths and their respective share in building up the adult gland explains the usual adult arrangement of the excretory system and its variations.

In the embryo of five weeks (Fig. 186) the two portions have grown in length. The dorsal or proximal outgrowth, developing between the layers of the mesoduodenum, is at this time the larger of the two, composed of a number of glandular vesicles clustered around the stalk represented by the parent duct.

FIG. 186.—Pancreatic buds of human embryo of five weeks. (Kollmann, after Hamburger.)

FIG. 187.—Pancreatic buds of human embryo of six weeks. (Kollmann, after Hamburger.)

The distal or ventral pancreatic growth, connected with the liver duct, is as yet small and presents only a few vesicular appendages. The duct of this portion empties in common with the hepatic duct into the duodenum.

In embryos of the sixth to seventh week (Fig. 187), the two glandular outgrowths have become connected with each other at a point which corresponds exactly to the divergence of the duct of Santorini from the main pancreatic duct (canal of Wirsung) in the adult gland (Fig. 188).

FIG. 188.—Human adult. Corrosion of pancreatic and common bile-ducts: ventral view. (Columbia University Museum, No. 1712.)

The secondary pancreatic duct (of Santorini) of the adult corresponds to that section of the proximal or larger embryonic outgrowth situated between the intestine and the point where the two glandular diverticula fuse with each other. Hence the canal of Wirsung in the adult is a compound product. It includes the duct system developed, in connection with the bile duct, in the head of the gland, forming the intestinal termination of the main duct. Its distal body portion on the other hand is derived from the duct system of the originally larger proximal outgrowth, including the entire peripheral portion which has become secondarily added to the duct of the ventral outgrowth to form together with it the canal of Wirsung. On the other hand the proximal portion of the duct system of this originally larger part becomes secondarily differentiated as the duct of Santorini.

Fig. 188 shows the normal adult arrangement of the pancreatic and biliary ducts in a corrosion preparation of the canal.

The duct of Santorini in this case opened by a separate orifice into the duodenum above the common opening of the biliary and pancreatic ducts (cf. p. 113).

Explanation of Adult Arrangement of Human Pancreatic Ducts and Their Variations Dependent Upon the Embryonic Development.—The smaller distal embryonic outgrowth is, as we have seen, from its inception in close connection with the duodenal end of the common bile-duct (Fig. 185).

The proximal outgrowth, situated nearer to pylorus and derived directly from the duodenal epithelium, is the larger and forms the greater part of the bulk of the adult pancreas (Figs. 186, 187).

FIGS. 189-192.—Series of schemata showing normal and variant adult types of biliary and pancreatic ducts.

FIG. 189.—Usual human adult type.

FIG. 190.—Persistence of early embryonal type.

FIG. 191.—Duct of Santorini has no duodenal orifice.

FIG. 192.—Duct of Santorini forms the only pancreatic duct. Separate duodenal openings of biliary and pancreatic ducts, resulting from failure of development of distal embryonal pancreatic bud.

If, notwithstanding this primitive arrangement, the distal duct (canal of Wirsung) appears as the main pancreatic duct in the adult, while the proximal (duct of Santorini) is secondary, this depends upon a union of the products of the two outgrowths in such a manner that the greater part of the duct system of the proximal and larger portion is transferred to the distal duct to form the adult canal of Wirsung, while the smaller segment of the proximal duct, between its opening into the duodenum and the point of fusion of the two outgrowths, forms the adult secondary duct of Santorini. This duct opens usually into the duodenum upon a small papilla situated about 2.5 cm. above the common duodenal termination of the bile-duct and canal of Wirsung (papilla Vateri) (Fig. 193). The duct of Santorini usually tapers toward the duodenal opening from its point of departure from the main duct, its caliber gradually diminishing in the direction indicated, so that it is smaller at the duodenal opening than at the point of confluence with the main duct (Fig. 189). Hence the secretion from the proximal head portion of the pancreas, conveyed by this duct and its tributaries, passes usually into the main pancreatic duct and not directly into the intestine through the duodenal opening of the duct of Santorini. The latter is, however, thus enabled to vicariously take upon itself the conduct of the pancreatic secretion in cases of obstruction or obliteration of the main duct (calculi, ulcers, cicatrices, etc.). In these cases of obstruction of the main duct the duct of Santorini enlarges and performs its functions.

Occasionally, without obstruction of the main duct, the duodenal opening of the duct of Santorini is large, and the flow of secretion evidently the reverse of the usual, *i. e.*, directly into the intestine.

In other cases, also without pathological conditions, the proximal duct is the larger of the two and serves as the principal channel of pancreatic secretion, the canal of Wirsung being small. This is evidently a persistence and further development of the early embryonic relative condition of the two outgrowths above described (Fig. 190). On the other hand the duct of Santorini may not open at all into the duodenum, terminating in small branches which drain the proximal part of the head of the gland (Fig. 191).

FIG. 193.—Mucous surface of human duodenum, showing entrance of biliary and pancreatic ducts and diverticulum Vateri. (Columbia University Museum, No. 1842.)

Schirmer has examined the arrangement of the pancreatic ducts in 105 specimens. In 56 of these the duct of Santorini passed from the main duct into the duodenum, opening upon a papilla situated 2.5 cm. above the common opening of the bile duct and canal of Wirsung.

In 19 the duct of Santorini was well developed but did not open into the duodenum.

In but 4 cases the duct of Santorini formed the only pancreatic duct, the lower opening being occupied by the bile duct alone (Fig. 192). We may assume in these cases failure of development of the distal outgrowth connected with the primitive hepatic bud, leaving only the proximal duodenal outgrowth to form the entire adult gland.

Figs. 188 and 189 show the normal arrangement of the duodenal openings of the biliary and pancreatic ducts.

Figs. 190 to 192 show schematically the variations in the relative development and the adult arrangement of the pancreatic ducts.

Diverticulum and Papilla Vateri.—From what has been said regarding the embryonic union of the distal pancreatic outgrowth with the hepatic bud it will be easy to recognize the corresponding features in the arrangement of the adult duodenal termination of the common bile-duct and canal of Wirsung. The dilated interior of the duodenal papilla (diverticulum Vateri) corresponds to the embryonic segment between the intestinal opening of the primitive liver duct and the point when this duct gives off the distal larger pancreatic outbud (Figs. 186, 187, 188, 193 and 194).

FIG. 194.—Adult human subject. Mucous membrane of pyloro-duodenal junction and of duodenum. (Columbia University Museum, No. 1840.)

FIG. 195.—Duodenum, with entrance of pancreatic and biliary ducts and well-developed diverticulum Vateri in the cassowary, *Casuarius casuarius.* (Columbia University Museum, No. 1821.)

The union of the pancreatic and biliary ducts to form the recess of the diverticulum Vateri, which then opens by a single common orifice into the duodenum, is better marked in some of the lower vertebrates than in man.

Fig. 195 shows the proximal portion of the duodenum of the cassowary (*Casuarius casuarius*) with the biliary and pancreatic ducts and the diverticulum at their confluence in section.

The development of these two main digestive glands as diverticula from the intestinal canal also explains the direct continuity of the mucous membrane of their ducts with that lining the duodenum, a fact which is of considerable importance in the pathological extension of mucous inflammations from the intestine to the duct system of the glands.

Development of the Pancreas in Lower Vertebrates.—In the embryo of the *sheep* two pancreatic buds are found, but the duct of the dorsal (proximal) outgrowth (duct of Santorini) subsequently fuses entirely with the main duct.

In the *cat* there are likewise two pancreatic outgrowths.

In the *chick* three pancreatic buds are visible about the fourth day.

Amphibia likewise present three embryonic pancreas buds.

The ventral (distal) outgrowth is double, the two portions proceeding symmetrically from each side of the hepatic duct. The single dorsal outgrowth is derived directly from the duodenal epithelium. Later on all these outgrowths fuse to form the single adult gland.

Fish also possess several (up to four) embryonic pancreatic outgrowths.

Recently in human embryos of 4.9 mm. cervico-coccygeal measure three pancreatic outgrowths have been observed, all entirely distinct from each other, one dorsal, budding from the epithelium of the primitive duodenum and two ventral, proceeding from the grooved gutter which represents the primitive ductus choledochus at this period. In embryos of from 6 to 10 mm. the two ventral outgrowths have already fused, hence only two buds, a single ventral and a dorsal, are now encountered.[4]

These observations place the development of the human pancreas in line with the triple pancreatic outgrowths, two ventral and one dorsal characteristic of the majority of the lower vertebrates, which have been hitherto carefully examined. The ventral or distal bud is probably double in the majority of vertebrates. The two segments fuse, however, so early that the derivation of the pancreas from a double outgrowth, as described above for the human embryo, practically obtains. In forms in which the adult gland presents a number of separate openings into the duodenum (cf. p. 118), the development would probably show multiple embryonic outgrowths from the intestinal hypoblast.

In any case the dorsal pancreatic bud appears to have developed in the vertebrate series before the ventral outgrowth and to be hence phylogenetically the older structure.

COMPARATIVE ANATOMY OF THE PANCREAS.

With the exception of *Amphioxus* and probably also of the *Cyclostomata*, the gland appears to be present in all vertebrates, varying, however, much in size, shape and relation to the intestinal tube. Usually it appears as an elongated, flattened, more or less distinctly lobulated organ, in close apposition to the duodenum between the layers of the mesoduodenum. In all forms in which the gland is found it is connected with the post-gastric intestine and marks the beginning of the midgut. In structure the gland is usually acinous, resembling the salivary glands. It is well developed in the selachians, forming a triangular body connected with the beginning of the midgut (Fig. 202). In some instances the gland elements do not extend beyond the intestine itself, but remain imbedded in the wall of the midgut, as in *Protopterus*. In certain adult teleosts the pancreas is surrounded by the liver (Fig. 196), in others it does not appear as a compact gland but is distributed in the form of finely scattered lobules throughout the mesentery between the two layers of this membrane. On account of this concealed position of the gland it was formerly believed that the adult teleosts did not possess a pancreas. The pyloric cæca (cf. p. 119) found in these forms were consequently considered to be homologous with the pancreas of the higher vertebrates.

FIG. 196.—A portion of alimentary canal of *Pleuronectes maculatus*, the flounder, with pancreas attached to biliary duct and concealed in the substance of the liver, which has been removed. (Columbia University Museum, No. 1491.)

FIG. 197.—Pancreas and biliary ducts of *Rana esculenta*, frog. (Wiedersheim, after Parker; both from Ecker.)

FIG. 198.—*Necturus maculatus*, mud puppy. Dissection of intestinal canal, liver, pancreas, and spleen, with blood-vessels injected. (Columbia University Museum, No. 1863.)

FIG. 199.—Pancreas and pancreatic ducts of rabbit. (Nuhn.)

FIG. 200.—Abdominal viscera of dog, showing arrangement of pancreatic ducts. (Nuhn.)

In *Myxinoids* a peculiar lobulated glandular organ is found imbedded in the peritoneal coat of the intestine near the entrance of the bile-duct, into which its lobules open separately. This organ possibly corresponds to the higher vertebrate pancreas.

An organ which may represent a dorsal pancreas is also developed in *Ammocœtes* (larva of *Petromyzon*), but its exact homology is still doubtful. It is possible that a true pancreas has not yet developed in the cyclostomata. In *Amphioxus* no trace of a pancreas is found. In all other vertebrates the gland is present. In certain amphibians, as the frog, the single pancreatic duct opens into the common bile duct (Fig. 197).

In lacertilians and in some chelonians a lateral offshoot of the pancreas is directed transversely and is adherent to the spleen. Fig. 113 shows the gland in *Chelydra serpentaria*. While the gland usually has a single duct, yet two ducts are found in a number of animals (many mammals, birds, chelonians and crocodiles). At times three ducts are encountered, as in the chicken and pigeon.

The arrangement of the pancreatic duct system among mammalia presents the following variations:

1. Mammals with *one* pancreatic duct, either connected with the bile-duct or entering the intestine independently:

Monkeys, most rodents (except the beaver), marsupials, carnivora (except dog and hyena), many ungulates (pig, peccary, hyrax, etc.), most ruminating artiodactyla.

(*a*) The pancreatic duct joins the common bile-duct before entering the duodenum in the monkeys, marsupials, carnivora, in the sheep, goat and camel.

The point of entrance of the combined duct into the intestine varies. In some forms it is near the pylorus, in others at some distance from the same. The common opening is situated 1½″ to 2″ beyond the pylorus in carnivora, and one foot behind the same point in the goat and sheep.

(*b*) The pancreatic duct does not join the bile-duct, but empties separately into the intestine, in most rodents and in the calf and pig.

In the calf the pancreatic duct opens into the duodenum 15′ beyond the bile-duct and 3′ beyond the pylorus.

In the pig the pancreatic opening is 5″–7″ beyond that of the bile-duct and 6″–8″ behind the pylorus.

2. Mammals with *two* pancreatic ducts, of which one usually joins the bile-duct: perissodactyla (except the ass according to Meckel), elephant, beaver, several carnivora, dog, hyena, and according to Bernard the cat. In the perissodactyla the proximal of the two pancreatic ducts empties, either combined with the bile-duct, or separate from it, but very close to it, 3″–4″ behind the pylorus. The second distal duct is smaller and opens several inches further down.

FIG. 201.—Section of dog's stomach, and proximal portion of duodenum, with entrance of biliary and pancreatic ducts. (Columbia University Museum, No. 1822.)

In most rodents the pancreatic entrance is placed at some distance from the pylorus. Fig. 199 shows the arrangement of the parts in the rabbit, in which animal the main distal pancreatic duct empties at a distance of 13″–14″ from the pylorus into the end of the duodenum, which intestine forms a very long loop, while the biliary duct, receiving the smaller proximal pancreatic duct, opens near the pylorus.

In the *beaver* the smaller proximal duct joins the bile-duct or even enters the duodenum anterior to the bile-duct, nearer the pylorus, while the distal larger pancreatic duct opens into the intestine 16″–18″ behind the biliary duct. Of the two ducts found in the dog (Fig. 200) the smaller proximal either joins the bile-duct or opens into the intestine close to it, 1″–1½″ beyond the pylorus. The larger distal duct opens into the duodenum 1″–1½″ behind the biliary duct. Fig. 201 shows the dog's stomach and proximal portion of the duodenum in section. The proximal smaller pancreatic duct here joins the biliary duct, and opens with it by a single orifice into the duodenum. The distal larger pancreatic duct opens independently into the intestine further caudad.

The parts in *Hyæna* present a similar arrangement.

Bernard always found *two* pancreatic ducts in the *cat*, one large principal duct and a second smaller accessory duct. Of these, the one situated nearest to the pylorus always united with the bile-duct. The pancreatic duct thus joining the bile-duct was sometimes the main duct, sometimes the accessory smaller duct.

Since the main function of the pancreatic juice is the conversion of starch into sugar, the gland appears better developed in general in herbivora than in carnivora, without, however, disappearing in the latter. In fact it is of considerable size in the carnivora, because the secretion also acts on the albuminous food substances and, though to a lesser degree, on the fats.

PYLORIC CÆCA OR APPENDICES.

In the *Cyclostomata* and *Selachians* the intestinal canal is in the main free from cæcal appendages, while a large portion of the tube is provided with a special fold of the mucous membrane which projects into the lumen of the gut (spiral valve). Fig. 43 shows the straight intestinal tract with the spiral valve of the longer distal segment in a cyclostome, *Petromyzon marinus* or lamprey. In Figs. 202 and 203 the selachian (shark) intestine is represented in two examples, while the similar spiral valve in a Dipnœan or lung fish, *Ceratodus*, is seen in Fig. 204.

FIG. 202.—Alimentary tract with spleen and pancreas of *Squalus acanthias*, the dog-fish. (Columbia University Museum, No. 1405.)

FIG. 203.—Alimentary canal of *Galeus canis*, dog-shark, in section, showing spiral intestinal valve. (Columbia University Museum, No. 1429.)

FIG. 204.—Alimentary canal with spiral valve of *Ceratodus forsteri*, the Australian lung-fish (Barramunda). (Columbia University Museum, No. 1645.)

On the other hand in the Ganoids and in many Teleosts longer or shorter finger-shaped diverticula of the midgut are found immediately beyond the pylorus in the region of the bile-duct.

These pouches or diverticula of the intestine form the so-called pyloric cæca or appendices of these fish. They vary very much in length, diameter and number in different forms.

Thus but a single diverticulum appears in *Polypterus* and *Ammodytes* (Fig. 205). *Rhombus maximus* and *Echelus conger* (Figs. 112 and 206) have two, and the same number appear in *Lophius piscatorius* (Fig. 207). Perca has three and the *Pleuronectidæ* have three to five.

FIG. 205.—Alimentary canal of *Polypterus bichir*. (Columbia University Museum, No. 1823.)

FIG. 206.—Alimentary tract of *Echelus conger*, Conger eel. Stomach, mid- and end-gut, liver, and spleen. (Columbia University Museum, No. 1430.)

FIG. 208.—*Pleuronectes maculatus*, window-pane. Stomach and mid-gut with pyloric cæca and hepatic duct. (Columbia University Museum, No. 1432.)

FIG. 207.—Stomach, duodenum, and pyloric cæca of *Lophius piscatorius*, angler. (Columbia University Museum, No. 1824.)

FIG. 210.—*Paralichthys dentatus*, summer flounder. Stomach and mid-gut with pyloric cæca and liver. (Columbia University Museum, No. 1431.)

FIG. 209.—*Pleuronectes maculatus*, window-pane. Stomach and mid-gut with pyloric cæca, in section. (Columbia University Museum, No. 1433.)

FIG. 211.—Pyloric cæca of *Gadus callarias*, codfish. (Columbia University Museum, No. 1825.) *A.* Bound together by connective tissue and blood-vessels.

B. Dissected to show confluence of cæca to form a smaller number of terminal tubes of larger calibre entering the intestine.

FIG. 212.—Alimentary canal of *Accipenser sturio*, sturgeon. Numerous pyloric cæca are bound together to form a gland-like organ. (Columbia University Museum, Nos. 1826, 1827, and 1828.)

The lower left-hand figure shows the mid- and end-gut in section, the latter provided with a spiral mucous valve.

Fig. 208 shows the stomach and the beginning of the midgut with four pyloric cæca in *Pleuronectes maculatus*, and Fig. 209 the same parts of this animal in section.

Fig. 210 shows the stomach and midgut of *Paralichthys dentatus*, the summer flounder, with three well-developed conical pyloric cæca. On the other hand in some forms the number of pyloric appendices is enormously increased, while their caliber diminishes. Thus 191 cæcal appendages are found surrounding the beginning of the midgut in *Scomber scomber*. A well-marked example of prolific development of the pyloric appendages is furnished by the common cod, *Gadus callarias* (Fig. 211). The appendices are in the natural condition bound together by connective tissue and blood vessels, so as to form a compact organ, resembling a gland (Fig. 211, A), and a similar arrangement is found in *Thynnus vulgaris* and *alalonga*, *Pelamys* and *Accipenser* (Fig. 212).

In the smaller upper figure on the left the stomach, mid-gut, and pyloric cæca are seen in section, showing the lumen of the latter and their openings into the mid-gut.

In some Teleosts (Siluroidea, Labroidea, Cyprinodontia, Plectognathi and Leptobranchiates) the appendices are entirely wanting. If there are not more than 8-10 appendices they usually surround the gut and empty into the same in a circle. In other cases they are arranged in a single line, or in a double row, opposite to each other (Fig. 213). Each appendix may open into the intestine independently, this especially where the number is limited and the individual pouches large (cf. Figs. 206-210), or several may unite to form a common duct.

Fig. 211, *B*, shows the appendices in *Gadus callarias*, the cod, freed by dissection from the investing connective and vascular tissue. It will be noticed that a considerable number of the tubes unite to form ducts of larger caliber which open into the intestine, as seen in the section shown in Fig. 214.

The pyloric appendices apparently have the same *significance* as the spiral intestinal fold of the Selachians, Cyclostomes and Dipnœans, *i. e.*, the production of an increase in the area of the digestive and absorbing surfaces of the intestinal mucous membrane. Hence, as stated, the appendices and the spiral fold are found to vary in inverse ratio to each other. Thus, for example, *Polypterus* (Fig. 205) still has a fairly well developed spiral fold and only a single pyloric appendix, while *Lepidosteus*, with but slightly developed spiral fold, has numerous appendices. It was formerly held that the pyloric cæca and the pancreas were mutually incompatible structures, and that where one is found the other will be wanting.

Hence the appendices were regarded as homologous with the pancreas of the higher forms. Recent observations have shown that this view is not strictly and entirely correct, while at the same time it merits consideration in several respects.

FIG. 213.—*Melanogrammus æglifinus*, haddock. Stomach, mid-gut, and pyloric cæca; spleen. (Columbia University Museum, No. 1598.)

FIG. 214.—Stomach and mid-gut of *Gadus callarias*, codfish, in section, showing intestinal openings of pyloric cæca. (Columbia University Museum, No. 1830.)

It is true that the pancreas in certain teleosts is now known to be present although concealed from observation in the liver or scattered in the form of small lobules between the layers of the mesentery (cf. p. 117), and that in a number of fish, such as *Salmo salar, Clupea harengus, Accipenser sturio*, both the appendices and the pancreas are encountered. Consequently these structures are not identical or even completely homologous, since they occur side by side in the same form.

On the other hand Krukenberg has demonstrated that the appendices pyloricæ may function physiologically as a pancreas by yielding a secretion which corresponds to the pancreatic juice in its digestive action. In the majority of forms, however, they apparently merely increase the intestinal absorbing surface, secreting only mucus.

These structures are nevertheless very interesting and instructive since they furnish a perfect gross morphological illustration of the embryonal stages just considered in connection with the development of the mammalian pancreas. In the adult ganoid or teleost these blind diverticula or pouches, varying greatly in shape, number and size, protrude from the intestine immediately beyond the pylorus, usually in close connection with the duodenal entrance of the bile-duct. Two or more of these pouches may unite to form a common duct or canal opening into the intestine.

These forms, therefore, offer direct and valuable morphological illustration of the manner in which the pancreas of the higher vertebrates develops, *i. e.*, as a set of hollow outgrowths or diverticula from the hypoblast of the primitive enteric tube. We can establish a consecutive series, beginning with forms in which only one or two diverticula are found, and extending to types in which the number of the little cylindrical pouches reaches nearly two hundred and in which they are bound together by connective tissue and blood vessels so as to closely resemble the structure of a glandular pancreas. This is one of the most striking instances in which the minute embryological stages of the higher types are directly illustrated by the permanent adult conditions found in the lower vertebrates. [The same statement, as we will see, holds good in reference to the development of the *liver*.]

RELATION OF THE PANCREAS TO THE PERITONEUM.

The gland becomes very intimately connected with the serous layers of the primitive dorsal mesentery. In order to clearly comprehend the adult serous relations it is necessary to make a distinction between two divisions or portions of the gland, based upon the altered relations of the primitive dorsal mesentery which result from the differentiation of the primitive simple intestinal tube into stomach and duodenum.

1. The primary outgrowth of the pancreatic tubules from the duodenum, *i. e.*, the part which is to form the "head" of the adult gland, is situated between the two layers of that division of the primitive dorsal mesentery which forms, after differentiation of stomach and small intestine, the *mesoduodenum*. Coincident with the rotation of the stomach, as we have seen, the duodenum and mesoduodenum exchange their original sagittal position in the median plane of the body for one to the right of the median line, balancing, so to speak, the extension of the stomach to the left (Fig. 218).

The original right layer of the mesoduodenum and the right surface of the duodenum now look dorsad and rest in contact with the parietal peritoneum investing the right abdominal background and the ventral surface of the right kidney and inferior vena cava. We have already seen that the descending portion of the duodenum in man becomes anchored in this position by adhesion of these apposed peritoneal surfaces. This fixation includes, of course, the structures situated between the layers of the mesoduodenum, *i. e.*, the head of the pancreas. Consequently, after rotation and adhesion, this portion of the gland turns one surface ventrad, invested by secondary parietal peritoneum, originally the left leaf of the free mesoduodenum, while the original right surface of the gland has become the dorsal and has lost its mesoduodenal investment by adhesion to the primary parietal peritoneum.

2. In order to understand the way in which the body and tail of the pancreas obtain their final peritoneal relations it is necessary to consider the development of the dorsal mesogastrium to form the omental bag. If we regard the primitive dorsal mesentery in the profile view from the left side (Fig. 215) it will be seen that, as already stated, the mesoduodenum is the first part of the membrane to be invaded by the pancreatic outgrowth from the intestine. Cephalad of the mesoduodenum the primitive dorsal mesogastrium (Fig. 215) is seen to protrude to the left and caudad to form, as already explained, the cavity of the omental bursa of the retrogastric space ("lesser peritoneal sac"). The further growth of the pancreas carries the developing gland from the district of the mesoduodenum into that portion of the dorsal mesogastrium which now forms the dorsal wall of the omental bursa (Fig. 216).

FIG. 215.—Cephalic segment of primitive mesentery in schematic profile view.

FIG. 216.—Schematic profile view of primitive mesenteries with formation of omental bursa and developing spleen and pancreas.

FIG. 217.—*Sos scrofa fœt.*, fœtal pig. Portions of thoracic and abdominal viscera hardened in situ. (Columbia University Museum, No. 1449.)

FIG. 218.—Schematic view of primitive mesentery after intestinal rotation and incipient formation of omental bursa from dorsal mesogastrium.

This double relation of the pancreas to the mesoduodenum and to the mesogastrium forming the omental bursa is well seen in fœtal pigs between two and three inches in length (Fig. 217).

The head portion of the pancreas is seen developing between the layers of the mesoduodenum, while the body and tail of the gland, extending to the left, grows between the two dorsal layers of the omentum bursa towards the spleen, which organ is found connected with the left and dorsal extremity of the omental sac derived from the dorsal mesogastrium.

Before the growth of the great omentum is pronounced the continuity of the mesoduodenum and dorsal mesogastrium can be readily appreciated (Fig. 218). But after the redundant growth of the membrane has carried the great omentum further caudad, the stomach and the two omental layers attached to the greater curvature lie in front of the structures included between the two dorsal layers and conceal them from view (Fig. 177).

FIGS. 219, 220.—Schematic transection of dorsal mesogastrium, pancreas, spleen, and stomach.

FIG. 219.—Before adhesion to primitive parietal peritoneum (arrow indicates the direction in which the adhesion takes place).

FIG. 220.—After adhesion and formation of secondary line of transition between mesogastrium and parietal peritoneum (lieno-renal ligament).

In sagittal sections to the left of the median line (Figs. 221 and 222) the pancreas now appears included between the layers of the great omentum near their point of departure from the vertebral column. (This point is of course identical with the prevertebral attachment of the primitive dorsal mesogastrium from which the omentum is developed.)

FIGS. 221, 222.—Schematic sagittal sections through stomach, pancreas, great omentum, and left kidney.
FIG. 221.—Before adhesion between dorsal and   FIG. 222.— mesogastrium and parietal peritoneum.   After adhesion.

The foregoing considerations will, therefore, lead to the conclusion that the pancreas presents, in regard to its peritoneal relations, two distinct segments:

1. The portion adjacent to duodenum (head and neck of the gland) is developed between the layers of the mesoduodenum.

2. The distal portion of the gland, comprising the body and tail, develops between the layers of the great omentum (dorsal segment), derived from the primitive dorsal mesogastrium.

The transections of the dorsal mesogastrium shown in Figs. 180 and 181 will now have to be amplified by the introduction of the body of the pancreas between the two layers of the vertebro-splenic segment, in addition to the splenic artery (Figs. 219 and 220).

Hence the following facts will be understood:

1. In the adult the splenic artery supplies a series of small branches to the pancreas as it courses along the cephalic border of the gland on its way to the spleen.

2. After the above-described adhesion of the original left leaf of the dorsal mesogastrium (vertebro-splenic segment) to the parietal peritoneum (Fig. 220), the dorsal surface of the body of the pancreas loses its peritoneal investment and becomes attached by connective tissue to the ventral surface of the left kidney.

3. The ventral surface of the body of the pancreas is in the adult lined by peritoneum of the "lesser sac"; in other words the organ has practically assumed a "retro-peritoneal" position, its ventral peritoneal covering appearing now as the dorsal parietal peritoneum of the retro-gastric space.

4. When completely developed the extreme end (tail) of the pancreas extends to the left, following the splenic artery, until it touches the mesal aspect of the spleen at the hilus.

5. If we, therefore, leave out of consideration for the moment the transverse colon and duodenum, which will be taken up presently, and confine ourselves to the arrangement of the stomach, pancreas and great omentum, a sagittal section to the left of the median line would result as shown in Fig. 222, after the adult condition of adhesion has been established.

The same process of fixation, which resulted in the anchoring of duodenum and head of pancreas, extends to the body of the gland and the investing omentum. The peritoneum lining the original left, now the dorsal surface of the gland, fuses with the primitive parietal peritoneum covering the diaphragm and the left kidney. The main body of the pancreas in the adult appears prismatic, giving a triangular sagittal section. The dorsal surface is adherent to the ventral surface of the left kidney; the ventral surface is covered by the secondary parietal peritoneum (original right layer of mesogastrium) which lines the dorsal wall of the retrogastric space and omental bursa (lesser peritoneal sac). The great omentum now appears to take its dorsal point of departure along the sharp margin which separates this ventral surface of the pancreas from a third narrower surface directed caudad. This surface, under the conditions which we are at present examining, would be lined by the peritoneum continued onto it from the dorsal layer of the great omentum. This peritoneum merges along the dorsal margin of this caudal surface of the pancreas with the general parietal peritoneum covering the left lumbar region and the caudal part of ventral surface of the left kidney. We have, therefore, along this line a secondary transition from visceral to parietal peritoneum, obtained by the obliteration of the original visceral peritoneum investing the dorsal surface of the pancreas before adhesion to the parietal peritoneum.

The pancreas assumes, therefore, in the adult a secondary retro-peritoneal position, covered on its ventral surface by peritoneum of the "lesser sac," while the caudal surface is lined by part of the general peritoneal membrane of the "greater sac." The dorsal surface, denuded of serous covering by obliteration, is adherent to the crura of the diaphragm, the aorta and the ventral surface of the left kidney.

It is now proper to compare the conclusions just derived from the study of the development of the human dorsal mesogastrium and connected structures (spleen and pancreas) with the conditions presented by the corresponding parts in one of the lower mammalia, which illustrate some of the human embryonal stages. Here again the abdominal cavity of the cat forms an instructive object of study.

The purpose of the following comparison should be twofold:

I. The mesogastrium, spleen and pancreas in the cat will clearly illustrate the process of human development above outlined.

II. The abdominal viscera of the cat, if properly arranged, will enable us to complete the consideration of this region by including the very important relations which the transverse colon and third portion of the duodenum bear in man to the great omentum and pancreas.

I. SPLEEN, PANCREAS AND GREAT OMENTUM OF CAT.

After opening the abdominal cavity it will be seen that the great omentum can be lifted up, exposing the subjacent coils of the small and large intestine, to which it adheres at no point. In other words the entire dorsal surface of that part of the original mesogastrium which forms the great omentum is free. It will be remembered that this is not the case in the adult human subject, because here the dorsal surface of the great omentum adheres to the transverse colon. Consequently in man only that portion of the dorsal surface of the omentum can be seen which extends between the transverse colon and the caudal free edge of the membrane.

It will be noted that on the left side the spleen is connected by its mesal surface to the omentum and through it with the stomach (gastro-splenic omentum). In other words the cat illustrates the human embryonal stage in which the spleen has appeared between the layers of the dorsal mesogastrium at the extreme left or blind end of the retrogastric pouch formed by the rotation of the stomach and elongation of the mesogastric membrane, but *before* the adhesion has taken place between the original *left* (now *dorsal*) layer of the vertebro-splenic segment of the mesogastrium and the primitive parietal peritoneum apposed to it (Fig. 219). Consequently the dorsal wall of the "lesser" sac in the cat is still composed of the two layers of the free vertebro-splenic segment of the mesogastrium, the primitive right (now ventral) layer not having been converted, as is the case in man, into secondary parietal peritoneum by adhesion of the original left (now dorsal) layer to the primitive prerenal parietal peritoneum.

If we now examine the relation of the pancreas to the peritoneum we can establish the following facts:

FIG. 223.—Abdominal viscera of cat, hardened and removed from body, showing relation of pancreas to mesoduodenum and dorsal mesogastrium, respectively. (Columbia University Museum, No. 728.)

1. The portion of the gland adjacent to the duodenum, corresponding to the "head" of the human organ, is included betweenthe two layers of the mesoduodenum. This membrane is free, so that the dorsal surface of this portion of the pancreas is seen to be invested by the dorsal layer of the mesoduodenum (Fig. 223). The duodenum and the mesoduodenum, the latter containing the head of the pancreas between its layers, can be turned toward the median line, so as to expose the entire ventral surface of the post-cava and right kidney. To illustrate the arrangement which is found in the adult human subject the descending duodenum and pancreas should be allowed to fall over to the right so as to cover the vena cava and the mesal part of the ventral surface of right kidney. The adult human condition will now be produced if we assume that the structures are fixed in this position by the obliteration of the apposed serous surfaces, viz., the parietal peritoneum over kidney and

vena cava on the one hand and the right layer of the mesoduodenum and the dorsal visceral peritoneum of the duodenum on the other.

2. In following out the pancreas of the cat in its entire extent, proceeding to the left of the pylorus, it will be seen that the body of the gland has extended between the two dorsal layers of the great omentum (primitive dorsal mesogastrium) over to the spleen (Fig. 223). Consequently the arrangement in the cat corresponds to the stage in the human development shown in Fig. 219 and Fig. 221 in which adhesion of the dorsal surface of the pancreas to the parietal peritoneum has not yet taken place.

It will be quite easy to reconstruct from the facts as demonstrated by the arrangement of the parts in the cat, the stage in the development of the lesser peritoneal sac in which the dorsal wall of the space is still formed by the proximal portion of the free dorsal mesogastrium (great omentum) and the structures included between its two layers.

It must then become apparent that the entire serous surface which in the adult human subject we regard as "parietal peritoneum of the lesser sac" lining the dorsal wall of the retrogastric space is derived from what originally was the right layer of the primitive sagittal dorsal mesogastrium.

II. RELATION OF GREAT OMENTUM TO TRANSVERSE COLON, TRANSVERSE MESOCOLON AND THIRD PART OF DUODENUM.

The second purpose to be accomplished by the study of the cat's abdominal cavity at this stage is the correct appreciation of the adult human conditions which are produced by areas of adhesion between the transverse colon, transverse mesocolon and third part of the duodenum on the one hand, and the dorsal mesogastrium, as great omentum, with the structures contained between its layers, on the other.

Perform the manipulations of the large and small intestine in the cat (see p. 67) which are required in order that the tract may be arranged so that it will correspond in general to the topographical conditions presented by the adult human subject. Locate the transverse colon and mesocolon and the third portion of the duodenum produced by these manipulations in imitation of the corresponding human structures. Then proceed to plot the different parts out successively as they would appear in a sagittal section (Fig. 224).

The following facts are to be noted and indicated on the plan of the section:

1. The great omentum is free, hanging down from the greater curvature of the stomach over the coils of intestine. Turning the omentum up it will be observed that the body of the pancreas is included between the two dorsal layers of the membrane.

2. The omentum, containing the pancreas, can be lifted up, exposing the next succeeding structure, viz., the transverse colon and mesocolon. In the cat the large intestine has been brought over, by the manipulations above indicated, into a transverse position so as to represent the human transverse colon and its mesocolon. It is therefore necessary to remember that in this mammal the fixation of the transverse mesocolon in the position indicated, by adhesion of ascending and descending mesocola to the parietal peritoneum of the abdominal background, has not yet occurred. Consequently the membrane must be held in the transverse position in order to represent the human arrangement.

FIG. 224.—Schematic sagittal section of abdominal viscera of cat, after the intestines have been rotated to correspond to the adult human disposition, to show lines of peritoneal reflection before adhesion.

FIG. 225.—The same figure indicating the areas of adhesion and peritoneal obliteration (shaded) which produce the arrangement of the adult human peritoneum.

1. Area of adhesion between opposed surfaces of great omentum and transverse mesocolon and colon.

2. Area of adhesion between parietal peritoneum, duodenum, and caudal layer of transverse mesocolon.

3. Adhesion of opposed walls of omental bursa leading to obliteration of distal portion of pouch and producing "gastro-colic" ligament of adult human subject.

It will of course be observed that both surfaces of the transverse mesocolon established in this way are free, not adherent to either omentum or pancreas on the one hand, nor to the transverse duodenum on the other.

3. The third or transverse portion of the duodenum is seen to be attached by the distal part of the mesoduodenum, both of the serous surfaces of the membrane being free. The duodenum having been brought from right to left transversely across vertebral column and aorta, underneath the superior mesenteric artery, the mesoduodenum, in the segment corresponding to the transverse duodenum, exchanges its original sagittal position for one in a horizontal plane, with cephalic (primitive left) and caudal (primitive right) surfaces.

Now compare the above arrangement of the intestines and peritoneum in the cat at once with the conditions presented in the adult human subject, reserving certain intermediate stages, as exhibited by some of the lower monkeys, for subsequent study.

The examination of a similar sagittal section representing schematically the adult human arrangement of the parts (Fig. 225) will reveal the following points of difference as compared with the cat:

1. The peritoneum covering the dorsal surface of the pancreas, derived from the primitive dorsal mesogastrium, has become adherent to the parietal peritoneum, as previously described.

2. The cephalic surfaces of the transverse colon and mesocolon fuse with the corresponding area of the dorsal (4th) layer of the great omentum (dorsal mesogastrium).

In the human fœtus in the 4th month the connection is still so slight that the omentum can readily be separated from the transverse colon and mesocolon.

Further dorsad the cephalic layer of the transverse mesocolon adheres to the serous investment of the caudal surface of the pancreas, derived, as we have seen, from the same dorsal layer of the great omentum.

3. The duodenum and mesoduodenum are fixed by adhesion on the one hand to the parietal peritoneum, on the other to the caudal layer of the transverse mesocolon near the root of that membrane.

4. The cavity of the omental bursa is usually obliterated in the adult caudad of the level of the transverse colon, by adhesion of the apposed surfaces of the two intermediate omental layers.

We have therefore three general areas of secondary peritoneal adhesion to deal with (Fig. 225), viz.:

1. Dorsal layer of primitive mesogastrium (great omentum) including the serous investment of the dorsal and caudal surfaces of the pancreas (Fig. 225, 1).	to	Parietal peritoneum, cephalic layer of transverse mesocolon and cephalic surface of transverse colon.
2. Transverse duodenum and mesoduodenum (Fig. 225, 2).	to	Parietal peritoneum and caudal layer of transverse mesocolon.

3. Between the apposed serous surfaces of the intermediate omental layers (Fig. 225, 3).

FIG. 226.—Schematic sagittal section of adult human peritoneum.

These areas of adhesion result naturally in the production of secondary lines of peritoneal transition as follows:

1. Figs. 225, 1; 226, 1, from the omentum, dorsal layer, to the caudal surface of transverse colon, caudal layer of transverse mesocolon and caudal surface of the pancreas.

2. Figs. 225, 2; 226, 2, from the caudal layer of the transverse mesocolon across the transverse portion of the duodenum to the parietal peritoneum and mesentery of the jejuno-ileum.

3. Figs. 225, 3; 226, 3, between the intermediate omental layers, forming the secondary caudal limit of the lesser sac.

These changes consequently result in the rearrangement of the adult human peritoneum in accordance with the following schema (Fig. 226):

We trace the peritoneum as the ventral or superficial layer of the great omentum from the greater curvature of the stomach caudad around the distal free edge of the omentum and

63

cephalad, as the dorsal layer, to the ventral border of the transverse colon. Here apparently this layer is continued across the caudal surface of the large intestine and beyond as the caudal layer of the transverse mesocolon. While this condition obtains practically in the adult it is to be remembered that the adhesion (at 1 in Fig. 225) prevents us from lifting the omentum away from the colon, and that consequently the apparent continuity of the dorsal layer of the great omentum with the caudal layer of the transverse mesocolon is the result of this peritoneal fusion.

Near the dorsal attachment or "root" of the transverse mesocolon the caudal layer of the membrane becomes continuous with the parietal peritoneum investing the transverse portion of the duodenum on its ventral aspect, which peritoneum in turn passes into the free mesentery of the jejuno-ileum (Fig. 225, 2). Comparison with the previous figures will show that we are dealing here with another area of secondary peritoneal fusion.

If we now open the "lesser peritoneal cavity" by dividing the two layers of the omentum attached to the greater curvature of the stomach (Figs. 225 and 226 in direction of arrow) we will apparently reach the upper or cephalic surface of the transverse mesocolon. This layer can be followed dorsad to the sharp border which separates the ventral and caudal surfaces of the pancreatic body and the membrane can be traced thence over the ventral surface of the gland to the diaphragm. (The connections with the liver and stomach shown schematically in the diagram (Fig. 225) are to be considered in detail subsequently.)

In the adult the peritoneal surface just described appears as the cephalic layer of the transverse mesocolon and its continuation dorsad. From the facts previously considered it will be at once apparent that we are really dealing here with a part of the third layer of the primitive omentum. We do not see the original cephalic layer of the transverse mesocolon. This membrane has become fused with the fourth omental layer, and its free serous surface obliterated in the stretch between the vertebral column and the transverse colon. Hence the human adult transverse mesocolon is apparently composed of *two* layers; the cephalic of these layers appears as peritoneum of the "lesser sac," in conformity with its derivation from the original third omental layer lining the interior of the omental bursa. The caudal layer, on the other hand, is a part of the general or "greater" peritoneal membrane. The entire adult transverse mesocolon, hence, comprises *four* peritoneal layers, of which only two remain as permanently free serous surfaces. These differ in their derivation, the cephalic layer being a part of the primitive dorsal mesogastrium (third omental layer), while the caudal layer is part of the primitive mesocolon. Between these two layers of the adult transverse mesocolon are included the two obliterated embryonic membranes, *viz.*, the fourth omental layer and the original dorsal layer of the transverse mesocolon.

Caudad the two layers of the adult transverse mesocolon surround the transverse colon and are continuous along the ventral margin of the intestine with the layers of the great omentum. Toward the vertebral column these layers again diverge. The cephalic layer, lining the "lesser peritoneal cavity" invests the ventral surface of the pancreas. The caudal layer continues over the caudal surface of the body of the gland and transverse portion of the duodenum into the parietal peritoneum and the free mesentery of the jejuno-ileum. Consequently the returning layers of the great omentum are said to surround the transverse colon and unite along the dorsal border of the intestine to form the transverse mesocolon, which membrane is continued dorsad toward the vertebral column as two layers. At the "root" of the transverse mesocolon these layers are then described as diverging, the cephalic passing up to line the ventral surface of the pancreas, while the caudal continues over the caudal surface of the pancreas and third portion of the duodenum into the parietal peritoneum and mesentery.

Wherever in this discussion of the transverse mesocolon the transition between the caudal layer of the membrane and the "parietal" peritoneum is referred to it is necessary to remember that this "parietal" peritoneum is the *secondary* investment of the abdominal background, formed by the surface of the ascending and descending mesocolon which remains free after the opposite surface and the vertical segments of the large intestine have been anchored by adhesion to the *primary* parietal peritoneum (cf. p. 81, Fig. 158).

A summary at this point of the course of the dorsal mesogastrium, in forming the great omentum and its subsequent connections, would show us that the membrane first

64

enlarges and descends towards the transverse colon (Fig. 177). The omental bag is formed by the descending or superficial segment (starting from the greater curvature of the stomach), turned toward the observer in the figure, and by the ascending or deep layer which is attached above to the dorsal abdominal wall, in front of the vertebral column and aorta along the original line of origin of the dorsal mesogastrium. Gradually growing and descending further, the deep segment becomes attached to the transverse colon. It also becomes connected, especially on the left side, with the diaphragmatic peritoneum (phrenicocolic lig.), so that its original starting point is no longer distinct. Finally the development of the spleen and pancreas between the layers of the dorsal segment and their subsequent connections obscure the original conditions.

Fig. 297 shows the primitive condition at a time when the connection with the transverse colon and mesocolon has not yet taken place.

The omental bag or bursa epiploica develops in the region of the dorsal mesogastrium and the viscera included between its layers, by changes in the position and extent of the membrane which finally result in placing a part of the right half of the primitive cœlom cavity behind the stomach. Up to the sixth week the line of origin of the dorsal mesogastrium is from the mid-dorsal line of the abdomen. It deviates from this origin to the left because the great curvature of the stomach to which it is attached turns in this direction. On this account, and because of the rapid growth of this portion of the mesogastrium, a bag or space is formed behind the stomach. The entrance into this space is situated to the right of the lesser curvature, behind the peritoneal layers connecting the same with the liver (lesser or gastro-hepatic omentum and hepato-duodenal ligament). The ventral wall of this space is formed by the dorsal surface of the stomach itself, the dorsal wall by the mesogastrium, turning to the left and presenting its original right surface, now directed ventrad. The caudal limit of the retro-gastric space is given by the turn of the mesogastrium to reach its attachment along the greater curvature of the stomach (rudiment of great omentum).

The stomach, in contributing to produce these changes, passes from the vertical to the oblique and finally into the transverse position. The pylorus, formerly directed caudad, passes up and to the right. The fundus develops and the original left side of the stomach becomes the ventral, the right side the dorsal. The original dorsal border, now the greater curvature, moving caudad, carries the attached dorsal mesogastrium with it into its new position. The mesogastrium now pouches to form the great omentum and rapidly enlarges. At first hardly projecting beyond the greater curvature, it increases in length until it forms a four-layered apron which hangs down as a loose sac over the transverse colon and the coils of the small intestine (Fig. 177). In the fœtus of six months the cavity of the omental bag extends caudad as far as the lower edge of the omentum. Later adhesions between the peritoneal surfaces lining the interior of the bursa limit this extension.

The omental bursa is therefore formed by a ventral lamella, consisting of two peritoneal layers, which hangs down from the greater curvature of the stomach and passes around the caudal free edge of the omentum into the double-layered dorsal lamella, which ascends, over the transverse colon, to the original starting point of the dorsal mesogastrium along the front of the vertebral column and aorta. Hence the "great omentum" is originally composed of four layers of peritoneum.

The dorsal double lamella becomes adherent over a considerable area to the parietal peritoneum of the dorsal abdominal wall. In this way the organs developed between the two layers of the lamella obtain their final fixed position. The pancreas becomes anchored and appears in the adult as a "retro-peritoneal" structure, while the spleen is attached by the "phrenico-lienal ligament" to the diaphragm.

In addition the dorsal omental lamella adheres in the fourth month to the cephalic layer of the transverse mesocolon and to the transverse colon.

Important illustrations of some of the intermediate stages in the human development of this portion of the peritoneal tract are afforded by the permanent adult conditions found in the abdominal cavity of some of the lower primates, notably certain of the cynomorphous monkeys.

FIG. 227.—Abdominal cavity of *Macacus rhesus*, Rhesus monkey, with the small intestine removed. (Columbia University Museum, No. 63/1831.)

Fig. 227 shows the abdominal cavity and disposition of the peritoneum in a macaque monkey (*Macacus rhesus*, ♂) in the ventral view, with the coils of small intestines removed and the omentum lifted up and reflected upon the ventral body wall. The following important points of difference from the arrangement in the *cat* on the one hand, and in *man* on the other, are to be noted:

1. The large intestine presents the typical primate course, with an ascending, transverse and descending colon. The ileo-cæcal junction is situated in the right iliac fossa.

2. The ascending and descending mesocola are still *free*, not having become adherent to the parietal peritoneum along the dorsal abdominal wall. Hence the caudal portions of the ventral surfaces of the two kidneys are still covered by the *primitive parietal peritoneum.*

3. The great omentum is not yet adherent to the transverse colon and mesocolon except for a short distance on the extreme right. At this point the dorsal layer of the omentum has begun to contract adhesions to the hepatic flexure of the colon and ascending colon, but the rest of the transverse colon is free. Differing from the human arrangement is a line of adhesion, uniformly present in these monkeys, between the dorsal surface of the omentum along its right edge and the ventral surface and right border of the *cæcum* and *ascending colon*, parts which normally are not adherent to the omentum in man.

4. Hence in tracing the omentum to the left of the limited adhesion to the hepatic flexure and ascending colon, *i. e.*, nearly throughout the entire extent of the transverse colon, we find the membrane passing freely without adhesion over the cephalic surface of the transverse mesocolon, which preserves its original free condition, independent of the omentum. This arrangement is shown in the schematic sagittal section in Fig. 230.

5. Tracing the omentum dorsad beyond the transverse colon and mesocolon the pancreas is reached. Here we encounter the first extensive area of omental or mesogastric adhesion. The omental peritoneum continues over the ventral and caudal surfaces of the gland, investing the same, but the dorsal surface has lost its serous covering and is anchored to the ventral surface of the left kidney. Hence a sagittal section would show the arrangement of the monkey's omentum as indicated in the schematic Figs. 229 and 230. Making now a general comparison of the peritoneal membrane of this animal with that of man, and of both with the preceding common embryonal condition, we can draw the following conclusions, indicated schematically in the five figures 228-232.

FIGS. 228-232.—Schematic sagittal sections of dorsal mesogastrium and omental bursa, in man, monkey, and cat.

FIG. 228.—Common embryonal condition, as illustrated by cat, after rotation and formation of omental bursa.

FIG. 229.—Area of adhesion between dorsal mesogastrium and primitive parietal peritoneum in *Macacus*, producing condition shown in Fig. 230.

FIG. 230.—Arrangement of great omentum as found in *Macacus rhesus*, shown without reference to areas of obliteration.

FIG. 231.—Corresponding section of human adult peritoneum showing, along dotted peritoneal lines, area of peritoneal adhesion.

FIG. 232.—Section showing human adult peritoneum without reference to area of adhesion.

1. The dorsal layer of the monkey's omentum in its proximal segment behaves in the same way as in man, *i. e.*, it becomes adherent to the primitive parietal peritoneum down as far as the caudal margin of the dorsal surface of the pancreas included between the primitive mesogastric layers forming by their further growth the omental apron.

Therefore we find, as in the human subject,

(*a*) The pancreas adherent to the ventral surface of the left kidney.

(*b*) A portion of the ventral surface of the kidney, cephalad of the pancreas, and the dorsal wall of the retrogastric (lesser peritoneal) space lined by secondary parietal peritoneum derived from the third layer of the omentum (original right layer of dorsal mesogastrium).

2. The monkey differs from adult man in the behavior of the dorsal omental layer in relation to the cephalic surface of the transverse mesocolon. The adhesion, which in the human subject fuses this layer with the transverse colon and mesocolon, does not occur in the monkey.

FIGS. 233-235.—Series of schematic sagittal sections through left kidney and adrenal, pancreas, and transverse colon, to show development of adult peritoneal relations.

FIG. 233.—Embryonic condition, as illustrated by cat, after rotation of intestine. Pancreas free between dorsal layers of great omentum. Transverse colon and mesocolon free. Kidney behind primitive parietal peritoneum.

FIG. 234.—Area of adhesion between: 1. Primitive parietal peritoneum. 2. Mesogastrium forming great omentum. 3. Colon and mesocolon.

FIG. 235.—Adult human arrangement, shown without reference to obliterated areas.

Hence we have in this animal the following conditions:

(a) The omentum is non-adherent to the transverse colon and transverse mesocolon.

(b) The caudal surface of the pancreas is lined by its original mesogastric peritoneum.

(c) The transverse mesocolon is formed by the original two layers of the primitive dorsal mesentery; hence its cephalic layer is not "peritoneum of the lesser sac" as is the case in man.

(d) The caudal part of the ventral surface of the left kidney below the pancreas, is covered by the original parietal peritoneum.

(e) Only one point or line of *secondary peritoneal transition* exists, where the dorsal layer of the omentum in the adult becomes continuous with the parietal peritoneum covering the caudal surface of the pancreas and the ventral surface of the left kidney.

Note: In the schematic sections shown in Figs. 228 to 232 the transverse colon is represented as far removed from the ventral surface of the left kidney, in order to make the peritoneal lines of the mesocolon more clear. Actually a sagittal section which would divide the kidney would cut the transverse colon at its extreme left end, where it turns close to the ventral surface of the left kidney and then follows its lateral border to form the splenic flexure (Fig. 235). The caudal part of the ventral surface of the left kidney in the adult human subject is covered by the peritoneum which, as secondary parietal peritoneum, is derived from the upper part of the right leaf (later ventral leaf) of the descending mesocolon. Hence it should be remembered that these diagrams present *combinations* of sections. A section which will show the full development of the transverse mesocolon is mesad of the kidney; while a section through the kidney would be too far laterad to show the transverse mesocolon.

Figs. 233, 234 and 235 show sagittal sections through the left kidney with the adult arrangement of the peritoneum and colon and the embryonic and adhesion stages leading to the same.

It will be observed that in all the schematic sections of the early embryonic stages the two layers of the transverse mesocolon are shown without dorsal attachment, as turning with the formation of a fold (Fig. 228 at x) into two layers descending ventrad of the parietal peritoneum. This is because the dorsal attachment of the mesocolon is at this stage still in the median line and would hence not be encountered by a sagittal section through the kidney, and because the two layers of the transverse mesocolon, immediately after rotation of the large intestine, are still directly continuous with the two layers of the descending mesocolon. That is to say, the cephalic layer of the transverse mesocolon is continuous with the dorsal (originally the left) layer of the descending mesocolon, and the caudal layer of the transverse mesocolon with the ventral (originally the right) layer of the descending mesocolon, which is, in the human subject, to assume subsequently the character of parietal peritoneum after the dorsal layer and the primitive parietal peritoneum have become obliterated by adhesion (Fig. 235).

Fig. 236 shows this continuity of the descending and transverse mesocolon as a permanent adult condition in the macaque. The fold of transition between the two is seen at x in Fig. 228. It will be noticed that the ventral surface of the left kidney, caudad of the adherent pancreas, is covered by the primitive parietal peritoneum, corresponding to section in Fig. 230.

RELATIONS OF SPLEEN AND OMENTUM IN *MACACUS RHESUS.*

The spleen in this animal has not contracted any extensive adhesions to the parietal peritoneum (the phrenico-lienal lig. of anthropotomy is not developed). It can be turned mesad so as to expose the lateral border and an adjacent segment of the ventral surface of the left kidney, as well as the dorsal surface of the tail of the pancreas at its tip, still covered by mesogastric peritoneum. Hence in the monkey the adhesion of the original vertebro-splenic segment of the mesogastrium, including the pancreas, to the primitive parietal peritoneum is less complete than in man.

MEDIAN ATTACHMENT OF DESCENDING MESOCOLON AND ITS RELATION
TO THE MESOCOLON OF THE SIGMOID FLEXURE IN THE *MACAQUE.*

FIG. 236.—Abdominal viscera of *Macacus cynomolgus*, Kra monkey. (Columbia University Museum, No. 1801.)

Fig. 236 shows the abdominal viscera, hardened in situ, of *Macacus cynomolgus*, the Kra monkey, in the ventral view and from the left side.

The great omentum is lifted up, the pancreas is adherent to the ventral surface of the left kidney, the caudal portion of which is covered by the primary parietal peritoneum, which can be exposed by turning the still free descending mesocolon mesad. The mesocolon retains its primitive attachment to the median line ventrad of the large prevertebral blood vessels. It is readily seen that adhesion between the left leaf of this free descending mesocolon and the parietal peritoneum down to the level of the iliac crest would produce the conditions found in the human adult, with an attached descending colon and a free sigmoid flexure; also that limited adhesion of the mesocolon of the sigmoid flexure to the parietal peritoneum would produce, as previously explained (cf. p. 97), the intersigmoid peritoneal fossa.

2. Ventral Mesogastrium and Liver.—The peritoneal reflections from the stomach to the liver, and the arrangement of the membrane in connection with the latter organ, remain for consideration.

Certain complicated adult conditions, encountered in this part of the abdominal cavity, make it desirable to arrange the subject for purposes of study under the following subdivisions:

I. The development of the liver and of its vascular system, and the significance of the adult circulation of the liver and of the fœtal remnants connected with the organ.

II. The anatomy of the ventral mesogastrium and the changes produced in the arrangement of the membrane by the development of the liver.

I. A. Development of the Liver.—The liver, like the pancreas, is developed from the duodenum as an outgrowth from the hypoblast lining the enteric tube. As we have previously noted, the first outgrowth of the hepatic diverticulum is closely associated with the distal pancreatic outbud; in fact the latter arises as a derivative from the hepatic duct rather than as a distinct outbud from the intestinal tube. (This close association of the hepatic duct with the pancreas is well seen in the arrangement of the concealed pancreas of some teleosts (cf. p. 117, Fig. 196).)

In point of time the liver is the first accessory structure to develop by budding from the primitive alimentary canal, the pancreas and lung following.

FIG. 237.—Longitudinal section of an embryo of *Petromyzon planeri*, four days old. (Minot, after Kupffer.)

In the primitive type of development, as seen in *Petromyzon* and in the Amphibia, the liver appears very early, as a diverticulum of the embryonic intestinal tube, near its cephalic extremity, projecting on the ventral aspect down into the mass of yolk-cells (Fig. 237). The short stretch of the primitive alimentary canal cephalad of the hepatic diverticulum corresponds to the foregut. With the development of the heart the primitive foregut becomes divided into pharynx and post-pharyngeal segment (œsophagus and stomach). The hepatic diverticulum then lies immediately dorsad of the caudal or venous extremity of the heart. Hence it is probable that the liver is an older organ in the ancestral history of the vertebrates than the pharynx or even the heart. The liver diverticulum lies in close connection with the omphalo-mesenteric veins which return the blood from the yolk-sac to the heart. In the course of further development, as will be seen below, the liver comes into very intimate relations with the venous circulation.

In human embryos of 3.2 mm. the primitive hepatic duct appears as a wide hollow pouch composed of hypoblast cells, growing between the two layers of the ventral mesogastrium, which membrane, extending between the ventral border of the primitive stomach and the ventral abdominal wall, will be subsequently considered in detail. The liver, in developing between the layers of the ventral mesogastrium, approaches very early the *septum transversum* or rudimentary diaphragm and becomes connected with the same. A mass of mesodermal cells, derived from the mesogastrium and from the primitive mesodermal intestinal wall surrounding the hypoblastic lining of the tube, covers the cæcal termination of the primitive hepatic duct, forming the so-called embryonic *hepatic ridge*. This mesodermal tissue accompanies the duct in its further growth and branching, forming the connective tissue envelope, known in the adult as the capsule of Glison. The primitive hepatic duct is directed cephalad in the mesogastrium between the vitelline duct and the stomach (Fig. 101).

In embryos measuring 4.25 mm. the duct is 0.24 mm. long. Later (in embryos of 8 mm.) the primitive single duct divides into two secondary branches, indicating, even at an early stage, the adult arrangement of the duct, as formed by the union of the right and left hepatic ducts (Fig. 185).

The gall-bladder in embryos of this size (8 mm.) is a well-defined cæcal diverticulum, branching caudad from the main hepatic duct.

The vesicular mucous surface is thus derived from the enteric hypoblast in the same way as the epithelial lining of the bile-ducts and capillaries. The external muscular and fibrous coats of the gall-bladder are developed from the mesoderm of the mesogastrium.

It is to be noted that at an early stage the gall-bladder is derived from the main duct close to the intestine, the latter duct being very short. Later on the common duct grows in length, making the liver more and more a gross anatomical organ distinct from the intestine. The cystic duct develops as the result of a similar increase in length of the cystic diverticulum. The two principal secondary branches of the hepatic duct give origin to sprouts or buds. These are derivatives of the hypoblastic cells of the larger ducts and may from the beginning be hollow, possessing a lumen continuous with that of the parent duct (Selachians, Amphibians). In warm-blooded animals these sprouts are at first solid, forming the s. c.*hepatic cylinders*, and only subsequently become hollowed out with the further development of the biliary duct system of the liver. The rapid growth of the organ leads to a great increase in the number of the hepatic cylinders. They spread out on all sides, finally coalescing with adjacent buds so as to form an interlacing network whose meshes are filled by blood vessels. After the hepatic cylinders have become canalized they preserve the same arrangement, hence the resulting biliary capillaries of the adult form an anastomosing network. Amphioxus and the amphibians have a single hepatic outgrowth (Fig. 49).

In the Selachians the liver arises as a ventral outgrowth at the hinder end of the foregut immediately in front of the vitelline duct, thus bringing the liver from the beginning into close proximity with the vitelline veins entering the heart. Almost as soon as formed the outgrowth develops two lateral diverticula, opening into a median canal. The two diverticula are the rudimentary lobes of the liver and the median canal uniting them is the rudiment of the common bile-duct and gall-bladder.

In the Teleosts the liver arises quite late (in the trout about the 25th day) as a solid outgrowth from the intestinal canal close to the heart. In the Amniota the liver arises in the same position as in the Anamnia, but, at least in birds and mammals, shows its bifurcation almost, if not quite, from the start. The two forks embrace between them the omphalo-mesenteric or vitelline veins just before they empty into the sinus venosus of the heart.

In the chick the liver appears between the 56th and 60th hour, the right fork being always of greater length but less diameter than the left. The hepatic outbud in the rabbit appears during the 10th day, and during the 11th day begins to send out branches.

In man, as above stated, the bud appears well marked in embryos of 3 mm.

[Certain adult variations make it appear possible that there are two human embryonic hepatic buds, a cranial and a caudal, as is the case in birds.]

I. B. Comparative Anatomy of the Liver.—The liver, phylogenetically a very old organ, occurs in all vertebrates, for the cæcal diverticulum of the intestine of amphioxus (Fig. 49) has probably the significance of a hepatic outbud.

The primitive form of the liver is symmetrically bilobed, a type which is seen well in the chelonian organ (Fig. 238).

FIG. 238.—*Pseudemys elegans*, pond turtle. Alimentary canal. (Columbia University Museum, No. 1437.)

FIG. 239.—Stomach, mid-gut, pancreas, and liver of*Boa constrictor*, boa. (Columbia University Museum, No. 1832.)

In size the liver is subject to great variations. It is usually larger in animals whose food contains much fat. Hence carnivora in general have a larger liver than herbivorous animals.

Its shape also varies considerably, depending on the form of the body cavity and on the amount and disposition of the available space. Hence in the snakes the organ appears long drawn out, flattened, almost ribbon-like (Fig. 239), while the relatively very large coronal diameter of the body cavity in the turtles permits the liver to expand transversely (Fig. 238).

FIG. 240.—Liver of*Macacus cynomolgus*, Kra monkey. (Columbia University Museum, No. 28/1833.)

FIG. 241.—Liver of *Pleuronectes maculatus*, flounder. (Columbia University Museum, No. 1679.)

In general, when the liver is large and the available space for its reception limited, it is usually split into several (two to seven) lobes, which permit, by mutual displacement, the accommodation of the organ to varying space-conditions of the body cavity (Fig. 240). Under the opposite circumstances, on the other hand, even the primitive bilobed character may disappear and the liver is then unlobed (Fig. 241).

The presence or absence of a gall-bladder depends apparently largely on the character of the food and on the habitual type of digestion. In many vertebrates digestion is carried on nearly continuously, without marked interruption, especially in many ungulates, ruminants and rodents. In such animals the gall-bladder is absent. It is also absent in several birds (most Parrots, Doves, Ostrich, Rhea americana, the Cuculidæ, Rhamphastos, etc.). This variability emphasizes the morphological fact that the biliary bladder is only a modified portion of the hepatic duct system, as shown by the development above outlined.

A great variety is observed in the arrangement of the biliary ducts, through which, at the period of intestinal digestion, bile passes from the liver and gall-bladder into the intestine, while in the intervals of digestion the secretion is only carried from the liver to the bladder. The following main types of the biliary duct system may be recognized:

FIG. 242.—Schema of hepatic and cystic ducts. (Nuhn.)

FIG. 243.—Schema of hepatic and cystic ducts. (Nuhn.)

FIG. 244.—Schema of hepatic and cystic ducts. (Nuhn.)

FIG. 245.—Schema of hepatic and cystic ducts. (Nuhn.)

1. The hepatic duct joins the cystic to form the common bile-duct, entering the duodenum by passing obliquely through the intestinal wall (Fig. 242). This form is encountered in man and in most mammals. It is also found in some birds (*Buceros*), many amphibians, and in some fish (*Lophius*). Instead of one hepatic duct two may join the cystic duct separately to form the common bile duct (*Phoca litorea*), or the number of hepatic ducts may be further increased. The separate hepatic ducts then unite successively with the cystic duct. This occurs in many mammals (as*Tarsius*, *Galeopithecus*, monotremes) and in some fishes (*Xiphias*, *Trigla*, *Accipenser*) (Fig. 243).

2. Of two hepatic ducts only one helps to form with the cystic duct the common duct, while the other leads from the liver transversely into the bladder, especially into the

neck, forming the hepatico-cystic duct (Fig. 244). This arrangement is found in several mammals (calf, sheep, dog).

3. No common bile-duct is formed. The hepatic and cystic ducts each empty separately into the intestine (hepato-enteric and cysto-enteric ducts), while a hepato-cystic duct carries the bile directly from the liver to the gall-bladder (Fig. 245).

Lutra vulgaris among mammalia, the majority of the birds and several reptilia present this type.

When the gall-bladder is absent a single large hepato-enteric duct is found, or instead a number of smaller ducts which enter the intestine successively.

I. C. Development of Vascular System of Liver.—In order to comprehend the peritoneal relations of the adult liver it is absolutely necessary to have a clear understanding of the development of the vascular system in connection with the gland.

For our purpose, in the first place, a serial consideration of the successive stages, illustrated by schematic diagrams, will prove most practicable. These diagrams represent the structures in the dorsal view, *i. e.*, in the position which they would occupy in the adult liver with the gland resting on its upper or convex surface and with the ventral sharp margin turned toward the beholder (see Fig. 259).

The development of the venous system, especially in connection with the liver, presents a somewhat complicated series of successive conditions. After having become familiar with the principal typical embryonal stages, as shown in the following diagrams, the student is strongly recommended to cement this knowledge by the comparative examination of the venous system. The permanent veins of the lower vertebrates, while in many cases not strictly homologous to those of the higher forms, yet are excellent objects for study, since they serve to illustrate temporary stages in the development of the mammalian venous system, and to that extent are of aid in comprehending one of the most difficult and important chapters in human anatomy. At the conclusion of the diagrammatic consideration of the mammalian development a number of comparative facts will be put together for this purpose.

FIG. 246.—Diagram of embryonic vascular system, without the portal circulation. (Parker, after Wiedersheim.) The dorsal aorta is formed by the junction of the right and left aortic roots arising from the confluence of the branchial arterial arches.

FIG. 247.—Diagram of the circulation of the yolk-sac at the end of the third day of incubation in the chick. (After Balfour.) The median portion of the first aortic arch has disappeared; but its proximal end forms the external, its distal the internal carotid arteries. The whole blastoderm has been removed from the egg and is viewed from below. Hence the left appears on the right, and *vice versa*.

Arteries in black.

Veins in outline.

1. Early Stage.—In the earlier developmental stages in mammalian embryos the primitive dorsal aorta extends caudad along the ventral aspect of the vertebral axis, giving off paired vitelline or omphalo-mesenteric arteries to the yolk-sac and allantoic arteries to the embryonic urinary bladder or allantois (Figs. 246 and 247).

The blood is returned from the vascular area of the yolk-sac by two vitelline or omphalo-mesenteric veins, which unite near the heart to form a common trunk, continued as the *sinus venosus* into the caudal or auricular extremity (venous end) of the primitive tubular heart (Figs. 246, 247 and 248).

2. Development of Allantois. Stage of Placental Circulation.—The placental circulation, replacing the temporary vitelline circulation of the earliest stages, is inaugurated by the appearance of two umbilical veins, which pass cephalad, imbedded in the tissue of the ventral mesogastrium, to empty into the sinus venosus near the vitelline veins (Fig. 249). The umbilical veins return the oxygenated blood from the placenta to the embryo. At first the right umbilical vein is the larger of the two.

FIG. 249.—Schema of umbilical veins, early stage.

FIG. 248.—Schema of

vitelline veins.

The sinus venosus at this time also receives two large veins, transversely directed, called the ducts of Cuvier, which are formed near the heart by the union of the anterior cardinal (primitive jugular) and posterior cardinal veins, draining respectively the head end of the embryo, and the body walls and Wolffian bodies.

The vitelline veins are placed on each side of the primitive small intestine, and become connected with each other by a broad anastomotic branch (Fig. 249). When the hepatic outgrowth buds from the duodenum the vitelline veins send out branches which break up into a wide-meshed capillary network in the mesodermic tissue enveloping the hepatic cylinders. Hence at this period the circulation in the vitelline veins is made up of three districts:

(*a*) Distal segment of veins, coursing along duodenum, and joined by a transverse anastomosis, before reaching the liver bud (subintestinal veins).

(*b*) Middle segment, from which capillary vessels are derived, ramifying upon and between the developing hepatic cylinders.

(*c*) Proximal segment, formed by the continuation of the proximal part of the vitelline veins into the sinus venosus of the heart.

FIG. 250.—Schema of primitive portal circulation.

3. Formation of Portal Circulation. A.—With the further development of the liver the direct connection of the distal segment of the vitelline veins with the sinus venosus becomes lost, the intermediate segment being entirely broken up into an intrahepatic network (Fig. 250). Hence all the blood brought to the liver by the vitelline veins (venæ hepaticæ advehentes) passes through the hepatic capillary circulation, before it is carried by the proximal segment of the vitelline veins (venæ hepaticæ revehentes) into the sinus venosus. The amount of this blood increases with new connections which the vitelline veins make with the venous radicles developing in the intestinal tract and its appendages. In proportion as, with the development of the placenta and reduction of the yolk-sac, the original significance of the vitelline veins as nutritive and respiratory vessels disappears, this secondary connection of the vitelline veins with the veins of the alimentary tract becomes more and more important, until finally the original vitelline veins, now properly called omphalo-mesenteric veins, return the blood from the intestinal tube, pancreas and spleen to the liver.

The venæ hepaticæ advehentes, becoming connected in this way with the developing intestine, pancreas and spleen, form the rudiments of the future portal system, while the venæ hepaticæ revehentes are prototypes of the hepatic veins of the adult circulation.

B. Development of the Portal Vein.—The distal subintestinal segments of the vitelline veins are early united by a transverse anastomotic branch. The section of the veins above this anastomosis is seen already in Fig. 250 to have assumed an annular shape, while the veins below the primary anastomosis are approaching each other to form a second ring-like junction.

FIG. 251.—Schema of further development of portal circulation and connection of same with umbilical veins in early stages.

FIG. 252.—Second stage in development of circulation through portal and umbilical veins. The proximal segment of the main portal vein is formed by the persistence of the left half of the distal and right half of the proximal periduodenal vascular ring of the omphalo-mesenteric veins. The distal segment of the main portal vein is the product of the fusion of the omphalo-mesenteric veins, and becomes connected with the veins of the intestinal canal, pancreas, and spleen. The proximal terminal segment of both umbilical veins becomes included in the system of the venæ hepaticæ revehentes.

FIG. 253.—Third stage in development of portal and umbilical veins during the placental period.

In Fig. 251 the subintestinal segments of the two vitelline veins are seen to have communicated with each other by transverse anastomotic branches around the duodenum, two of these branches being situated ventrad and one dorsad of the intestinal tube. These branches, and the portions of the primitive vitelline veins between their points of derivation, form two vascular loops or rings, encircling the primitive duodenum (Fig. 251).

The distal portions of the vitelline veins, before reaching the caudal annular duodenal anastomosis, next fuse into a single longitudinal vessel which also receives the veins from the stomach, intestine, spleen, and pancreas, and forms the beginning of the portal vein.

By atrophy of the right half of the lower, and of the left half of the upper duodenal venous ring (Figs. 252 and 253), the proximal portion of the portal vein is formed as a single vessel, taking a spiral course around the duodenum (Fig. 256). Hence in theadult the portal vein and its principal branch (the superior mesenteric vein) crosses over the ventral surface of the duodenum (third portion), turns along the mesal side of the second portion, and then continues to the liver along the dorsal aspect of the first portion (Fig. 254). *Note*—In comparing Fig. 254with the schematic figures it should be noted that the same presents the parts in the *ventral* view, while the schemata offer the *dorsal*aspect.

4. Changes Leading to the Final Arrangement of the Umbilical Veins.—A very important rearrangement of the umbilical veins takes place. These veins originally course in the lateral abdominal wall, close to the fold of the amnion (Fig. 255), and then turn cephalad of the developing liver along the septum transversum to empty into the sinus venosus at each end (Figs. 249 and250). The right umbilical vein is at first the larger.

This symmetrical arrangement, and the direct connection of the umbilical veins with the sinus venosus, now becomes lost by the occurrence of the following changes:

1. At first (Fig. 249) all the blood carried to the liver by the omphalo-mesenteric veins passes through the hepatic capillary network before being conducted by the venæ revehentes to the sinus venosus. Very early, however, a new intrahepatic channel develops, the ductus venosus (Figs. 250-253), which passes obliquely between the entrance of the left omphalo-mesenteric vein into the capillary system (l. v. advehens) and the termination of the right omphalo-mesenteric vein (r. vena revehens) in the sinus venosus.

In human embryos of 4 mm. the ductus venosus can already be distinguished, and in embryos of 5 mm. the vessel has assumed considerable proportions.

2. A communication is next established on both sides between the capillary hepatic network in the portion of the liver nearest to the abdominal wall and the umbilical veins as they ascend imbedded in the abdominal wall (Fig. 251).

This connection is usually from the start larger on the left side and connects with the left omphalo-mesenteric vein just at the point where the same is about to be continued into the ductus venosus. This connection becomes rapidly larger, so that the ductus venosus, which at first appeared merely as an anastomotic channel between the left omphalo-mesenteric vein and the terminal portion of the right omphalo-mesenteric vein, now forms the main continuation of the left umbilical vein. This vessel grows very rapidly up to its connection with the ductus venosus and soon exceeds the right umbilical vein in size (Fig. 252). Beyond the ductus venosus on the other hand the proximal segment of the left umbilical vein diminishes in size, and loses its independent character by incorporation in the hepatic circulation. Only its terminal portion, emptying into the sinus venosus, is preserved. This is surrounded by the growing masses of hepatic cylinders and is converted into a vena revehens.

The connection of the right umbilical vein with the liver vessels is at first symmetrical to that on the left side, but less strongly developed. The effect of this connection is to reduce in the same way the proximal segment of the right umbilical vein and to convert its termination into a vena revehens. With the great development of the left vein, however, the vein on the right side gradually diminishes and finally loses its connection with the intrahepatic circulation altogether. The right umbilical vein is now reduced to a vessel of the ventral abdominal wall, which carries blood in the reverse of the original direction, *i. e.*, from the abdominal wall caudad *into* the left umbilical vein (Figs. 253 and 255).

The connection thus established between the umbilical vein and the portal circulation results in the formation of a single large (the original left) umbilical vein which, throughout the remainder of fœtal life, returns all of the placental blood (Fig. 253).

The newly developed hepatic portion of the left umbilical vein becomes, however, not only connected with the ductus venosus, but also with the right part of the upper venous ring, derived from the right omphalo-mesenteric vein (Fig. 253). This connection forms the left portal vein of the adult, and enlarges rapidly.

FIG. 254.—Corrosion preparation showing course of portal vein and tributaries in relation to duodenum. (Columbia University Museum, No. 1857.)

FIG. 255.—Human embryo of 10 mm. cervico-coccygeal measure. Heart and ventral body-wall removed to show sinus venosus and entering veins. (Kollmann, after His.)

The terminations of the ductus venosus and of the venæ hepaticæ revehentes undergo a number of secondary changes in relative position. The left hepatic vein loses its direct connection with the sinus venosus, and now opens into the termination of the ductus venosus, into which the right hepatic vein also empties. This common vessel (v. hepatica communis) subsequently forms the proximal segment of the postcava when this vessel develops (Fig. 256).

FIG. 256.—Final stage of development of portal and umbilical veins in the placental period.

FIG. 257.—Schema of relation of postcava to hepatic veins and ductus venosus.

The blood, therefore, returned to the liver by the left umbilical vein divides at the transverse fissure into three streams. Two of these pass through the connection with the portal vein and through branches developed from the hepatic part of the umbilical vein into the capillary system of the right and left lobe. The third continues through the ductus venosus to the common hepatic vein and sinus venosus (Fig. 256). The ductus venosus thus becomes the chief vessel returning arterialized placental blood to the heart. When the postcava develops fully the hepatic segment of this vessel also joins the terminal part of the ductus venosus (Fig. 256) and gradually replaces the same as the main returning venous channel, the proximal part of the ductus venosus being incorporated in the vena cava (Fig. 257). The postcava then receives the right hepatic veins separately, while the left hepatic veins and ductus venosus open together into the main vein. This condition obtains up to the time of birth and the consequent interruption of the placental circulation.

While at first the ductus venosus communicates throughout its entire length with the meshwork of the hepatic capillary system, a separation into two segments, i. e., ductus venosus proper and intrahepatic segment of umbilical vein, is established after the free communication with the left umbilical vein takes place. This condition is exhibited in Fig. 258, which represents the corroded venous system of the fœtal liver, and in Fig. 259, showing an injected liver in the fœtus at term.

FIG. 258.—Corrosion preparation of venous system of human liver in fœtus at term. (Columbia University Museum, No. 1834.)

FIG. 259.—Injected and hardened human liver from fœtus at term. (Columbia University Museum, No. 1853.)

FIG. 260.—Diagram of intrahepatic fœtal venous circulation.

FIG. 261.—Diagram illustrating the changes in the intrahepatic venous circulation resulting from the cessation of the placental circulation at birth.

It will be observed that the umbilical vein on entering the liver gives off a large branch to the left lobe, and a smaller branch on the right side to the quadrate lobe, which act as the main venæ advehentes of these portions of the liver. Arrived at the transverse fissure the umbilical vein divides into three branches, at right angles to each other. The left branch enters the left lobe, the right branch becomes directly continuous with the left main division of the portal vein, while the central branch, continuing the direction of the umbilical vein, passes dorsad, as the ductus venosus proper, to join the left hepatic vein close to its entrance into the postcava.

5. Changes Consequent upon the Establishment of Pulmonary Respiration.—
After birth the umbilical vein and its continuation, the ductus venosus, become obliterated, the former constituting the round ligament of the liver, the latter the ligament of the ductus venosus, both structures imbedded in corresponding portions of the sagittal fissure on the

74

caudal and dorsal surfaces of the adult liver (Figs. 284 and 286). The lateral branches of the umbilical vein, however, in its course from the ventral margin of the liver to the transverse fissure (Fig. 258), remain pervious and are transferred to the portal circulation.

It will be noticed, in reference to the *direction* of the blood current, that at birth a sudden reversal takes place in the right terminal branch of the umbilical vein at the transverse fissure (Figs. 260 and 261). Before birth the blood current of the umbilical vein divides into three streams, right, left and central. The latter enters the ductus venosus. The left enters the liver directly, the right traverses, from left to right, the segment between the termination of the umbilical and the bifurcation of the portal vein. This segment in the adult carries blood from right to left, as left branch of the portal vein. In the fœtus, however, the blood traverses this segment from left to right, in passing from the umbilical to the right branch of the portal vein. The blood entering the liver through the portal vein passes chiefly into the right division of that vessel (Fig. 260).

After birth all the venous blood entering the liver passes through the portal vein. In the right division the direction of the current is the same as in the fœtus.

On the left side, however, the current is now from right to left, from the bifurcation of the portal into the channels of the left lobe formerly connected with the umbilical vein (Fig. 261).

Hence the direction of the current in this segment is reversed at birth.

SUMMARY OF HEPATIC CIRCULATION.

The foregoing consideration of the development shows us that the hepatic circulation presents successively three main stages:

1. Omphalo-mesenteric or Vitelline Stage, which results in the laying down of the primary capillary circulation of the liver and in the establishment of its connection with the developing veins of the alimentary tract (primitive portal channels).

2. Umbilical or Placental Stage, in which the greater part of the blood circulating through the liver is oxygenated blood returned from the placenta by the umbilical vein, accounting for the rapid growth and relatively large size of the organ during fœtal life.

The placental blood uses the preformed capillary channels of the vitelline or primitive portal system in the liver, and the same rapidly extend and enlarge with the accelerated growth of the gland. During this stage venous blood is also returned from the alimentary tract to the liver by the portal vein, produced by fusion of the distal segments of the primitive vitelline veins and their secondary connection with the mesenteric, splenic and pancreatic veins (omphalo-mesenteric development of primitive vitelline veins).

3. Adult or Portal Stage.—With the interruption of the placental circulation the portal vein assumes again its original position as the only vein carrying blood to the liver. With the establishment of intestinal digestion and absorption this vessel grows rapidly in size.

COMPARATIVE ANATOMY OF THE HEPATIC VENOUS CIRCULATION.

For the purpose of fixing the main facts in connection with the development of the higher mammalian hepatic circulation, and in order to obtain a demonstration of the cycle through which the different veins pass, the student is recommended to examine, preferably by personal dissection, a limited series of lower vertebrates which can be readily procured and easily injected. The following series has been selected, but it will be understood that other forms can be substituted, according to the local conditions which govern the supply of the material.

    1. *Fish.* A *Selachian*, the common skate (*Raja ocellata*) or dog-fish (*Acanthias vulgaris*).

    2. *Amphibian.*

(*a*)   Urodele. *Necturus*   *maculatus.*
(*b*) Anura. The common *frog.*

    3. *Reptile.*

Preferably, on account of the ease of injection, one of the larger lizards, as *Iguana tuberculata.* The turtles, although somewhat more difficult objects to prepare, can be substituted.

    4. *Bird.* The common fowl.

    5. Human fœtus at term.

1. Fish.—The venous system can be injected by tying a canula in the lateral vein, and injecting both cephalad and caudad, or by injecting cephalad through the caudal vein. The injection of the systemic veins can also be made caudad through one of the ducts of Cuvier, combined with an injection cephalad of the caudal vein.

FIG. 262.—Diagram of the veins of a selachian. (Wiedersheim, after Parker.)

The lateral vein arises from a venous network surrounding the cloaca, receiving one or more cutaneous veins of the tail, veins of the body-wall, and veins of the pelvic fins.

The caudal vein divides at the posterior end of the kidney into the two renal-portal veins, from which the advehent veins of the renal-portal system are derived. The revehent renal-portal veins join to form the posterior cardinal veins, which, after dilating enormously to form the cardinal sinuses, join with the anterior jugular, subclavian, and lateral veins to form the ducts of Cuvier. The latter receive the inferior jugular veins, from the deep parts of the head and neck and the terminations of the hepatic portal system (hepatic sinus).

The hepatic portal vein is formed by the veins of the œsophagus, stomach, and intestines. After traversing the capillary vessels of the liver, the revehent hepatic veins unite to form an extensive hepatic sinus before entering the heart.

The following main facts are to be noted in the venous system of the Selachian (Fig. 262):

1. There are Two Portal Systems.(*a*) *Renal Portal System.*—The caudal vein divides near the vent into two branches which course along the lateral border of the kidneys, sending *afferent* or*advehent* veins into the organ. The blood traverses the renal capillaries and is gathered together by the*efferent* or*revehent* veins, which empty into median paired vessels, the posterior cardinals.

(*b*) *Hepatic Portal System.*—The veins of the digestive tract and appendages unite to form a hepatic portal vein. The blood after traversing the capillary system of the liver is collected by hepatic veins, which form a dilated hepatic sinus emptying into the sinus venosus of the heart.

2. The middle segment of the intestine, presenting a spiral valve in the interior, gives rise to a vein emptying into the portal vein which corresponds to the subintestinal vitelline vein of the mammalian embryo (Fig. 202).

3. The posterior cardinal veins, also greatly dilated and forming the posterior cardinal sinus, join, near the heart, the veins returning blood from the head, the anterior cardinal or jugular, to form a transversely directed trunk, the duct of Cuvier, which empties into the sinus venosus at the auricular extremity of the heart. Into the duct of Cuvier empties on each side a *lateral vein* returning the blood from the body walls. This vein can be considered, for our present purpose, as representing in general the abdominal vein of amphibians and reptiles, and the umbilical vein of the mammalian embryo.

The adult selachian venous system is therefore to be considered as illustrating the following conditions above encountered in our study of the embryology of the mammalian venous system.

1. The heart illustrates excellently the stage in the mammalian development, in which auricular and ventricular segments have differentiated, but before the division of the cavities into a pulmonary and systemic portion by the development of the auricular and ventricular septa and the division of the arterial trunk into pulmonary artery and aorta.

The sinus venosus still exists, as an ante-chamber to the auricular cavity proper, receiving on each side the ducts of Cuvier, which represent the fusion product of the systemic veins, anterior and posterior cardinal.

2. The hepatic portal circulation corresponds to the mammalian stage in which the vitelline veins have become omphalo-mesenteric by joining the intestinal veins.

The spiral vein remains as a portion of the original vitelline vein corresponding to the subintestinal segment of the mammalian embryo (cf. Figs. 248 and 249).

The selachian portal vein represents the united vitelline veins, into which the veins of the digestive tract open.

In the liver we find a simple system of venæ advehentes, derived from the branching of the portal vein, a hepatic capillary network, and venæ revehentes, the proximal remnants of the original vitelline veins which carry the liver blood to the sinus venosus. The condition of the hepatic circulation corresponds therefore to the stage shown in Fig. 250 of the mammalian development. There is as yet no association of the hepatic venous system with the representative of the umbilical vein (the lateral vein of the selachian).

FIG. 263.—Diagram of the veins of urodele amphibian (*Salamandra maculosa*). (Wiedersheim.)

The caudal vein bifurcates at the posterior extremity of the kidneys to form the afferent trunks of the renal-portal system along the lateral border of the kidneys, from which the advehent veins of the renal-portal system are derived. The iliac or femoral vein divides into an anterior and a posterior branch, the latter opening into the afferent renal-portal vein, while the former, uniting with the one of the opposite side, forms the abdominal vein, and receives vessels from the bladder, cloaca, and end-gut. The revehent veins of the renal-portal system, emerging upon the ventral surface of the kidneys, empty into a single median vessel, the distal or renal section of the postcava or vena cava inferior. Proceeding cephalad, the proximal or hepatic section of this vessel, after traversing the liver and receiving the revehent hepatic veins of the hepatic portal system, empties into the sinus venosus of the heart. Previous to entering the liver the postcava gives off the two posterior cardinal or azygos veins, which continue cephalad, receiving tributary segmental veins from the body-walls and reach the sinus venosus by joining the subclavian veins. These latter uniting with the anterior cardinal (jugular) veins form the ducts of Cuvier (precaval veins).

The abdominal vein continues cephalad in the ventral mesogastrium to the liver, giving off a number of smaller branches, which enter the hepatic portal circulation by penetrating the ventral surface of the liver between the layers of the ventral mesogastrium, while the main continuation of the vessel joins the hepatic portal vein at its point of entrance into the liver.

The hepatic portal vein is formed by tributaries returning the blood from the digestive tract (intestinal canal, spleen, pancreas). The blood, after traversing the hepatic portal circulation, is conducted by the hepatic revehent veins to the proximal section of the postcava. A number of secondary or accessory portal veins pass from the anterior portion of the intestinal canal (œsophagus, stomach) directly to the liver.

FIG. 264.—Dissection of veins of *Necturus maculatus*, mud-puppy. (Columbia University Museum, No. 1835.)

The postcava has been divided at the cephalic end of the liver just before entering the sinus venosus, and the postcardinals have been cut prior to their junction with the subclavian veins.

The stomach has been turned caudad. The abdominal vein has been divided after the common trunk has been formed by branches from the iliac veins. The latter are seen entering the afferent renal-portal vein, derived from the bifurcation of the caudal vein, along the lateral border of the kidneys.

The junction of the main trunk of the abdominal vein with the hepatic portal vein takes place close to the liver under cover of the pancreas. A series of accessory portal veins continuous with the abdominal vein enter the ventral surface of the liver between the layers of the ventral mesogastrium. The inter-renal segment of the postcava receives the revehent renal-portal veins. The iliac vein enters the advehent renal-portal veins derived from the caudal vein.

FIG. 265.—Venous system of *Rana esculenta*, frog. (Ecker.)

3. The lateral veins, which we can, as stated, regard for purposes of illustration, without prejudging their genetic significance, as representing the mammalian embryonic umbilical veins, still present the condition corresponding to the early mammalian embryonal stage shown in Fig. 250. They are veins of the body walls, emptying cephalad of the liver, directly into the ducts of Cuvier, and through them into the sinus venosus of the heart.

Fig. 262 shows the arrangement of the venous system in a typical selachian diagrammatically.

2. Amphibian. (*a*) Urodele.—The following points are to be noted in comparison with the preceding form:

1. The two ducts of Cuvier entering into the sinus venosus are formed by the anterior cardinal and subclavian veins, which latter, having appeared with the full development of an

77

anterior extremity, receives the posterior cardinal veins, representing the mammalian azygos system.

2. The renal portal circulation persists. The caudal vein is, however, no longer the only afferent vein of this system. With the full development of a posterior extremity an iliac vein returns the blood from the same and gives a large branch (afferent to the portal renal system), while the trunk continues cephalad as an anterior abdominal vein, corresponding to the lateral selachian vein, emptying in the hepatic portal vein.

3. The efferent veins of the renal portal system no longer unite to form the posterior cardinal, as in the Selachian, but empty into a new median vessel, the inferior vena cava, or postcava, which has replaced the distal segments of the posterior cardinal veins.

The postcava now carries the blood from the kidneys directly to the heart. The original posterior cardinal veins still persist in their proximal segments, as smaller trunks connecting the distal part of the postcava with the ducts of Cuvier through the subclavian veins. The ducts of Cuvier represent the precavæ (venæ cavæ superiores) of mammalia and the postcardinals the mammalian azygos veins.

4. The hepatic portal system differs in two respects from the Selachian type.

(*a*) The blood returned to the liver from the digestive tract by the portal vein becomes mixed before entering the gland with the blood returned from the posterior extremities and abdominal walls by the abdominal vein.

This vein, paired below and continuous with the lateral of the two branches into which the iliac vein divides, becomes united into a single trunk above and empties into the portal vein.

The abdominal vein represents the lateral vein of the Selachian and corresponds to the umbilical vein of the higher vertebrates.

(*b*) The venæ hepaticæ revehentes do not empty directly into the sinus venosus, but into the proximal portion of the postcava.

Hence the adult urodele venous system illustrates, in reference to the mammalian development, these stages:

1. The umbilical (abdominal) vein has lost its direct connection with the sinus venosus. The proximal segment, cephalad of the liver, has disappeared, and its blood now passes directly into the hepatic circulation by its union with the portal vein.

(Cf. stage schema Figs. 251 and 252.)

2. The postcaval vein has made its appearance, largely replacing the posterior cardinal veins, whose proximal segments became converted into secondary vessels (azygos) uniting the system of the postcava with that of the duct of Cuvier (mammalian præcava), while their distal segments are transformed into the distal portion of the postcava.

The postcava, therefore, is made up of two districts:

(*a*) The proximal portion is a new vessel, developed in connection with the hepatic venous system.

(*b*) The distal portion is derived from the distal segments of the original posterior cardinal veins.

The termination of the hepatic veins in the postcava corresponds to the stage shown in schema Fig. 256.

Fig. 263 gives a schematic representation of the arrangement of the venous system in a typical urodele amphibian (*Salamandra maculosa*).

In Fig. 264 the dissected venous system of *Necturus maculatus*, the mud puppy, is shown in an injected preparation.

(*b*) **Anure.**—The venous system of *Rana esculenta* is shown in Fig. 265. Comparison with venous system of *urodele*:

1. The abdominal vein, corresponding to the mammalian umbilical vein, has assumed a greater importance in reference to the hepatic circulation. It is a large trunk, continuous below with the pelvic vein, terminating above in two branches, which enter the liver as afferent veins, being joined just prior to the division by the hepatic portal vein.

2. A small cardiac vein, coming from the heart, empties into the angle of bifurcation of the abdominal vein.

3. The postcava is well developed, formed by large efferent renal veins. It entirely replaces the posterior cardinal veins which are absent in the adult animal.

4. A right and left præcaval vein is formed by the union of two jugular trunks with the vein of the anterior extremity and a large musculo-cutaneous vein.

Comparison with the mammalian development: the venous system of this amphibian can be used to illustrate the mammalian embryonal stage shown in schema Fig. 252, in which the abdominal or umbilical vein has become the most important vessel in the afferent hepatic venous system.

The communication existing by means of the cardiac vein between the heart and the hepatic afferent system may suggest, but *purely for illustrative purposes*, the direct connection of the umbilical vein with the heart by the ductus venosus in the mammalian embryo (cf. schema Figs. 250-256).

3. Reptile.—In *Iguana* the renal portal system is well developed. The caudal vein, returning the blood from the tail and the cavernous tissue of the genital organs, continues for a short distance upon the fused caudal end of the two kidneys (Fig. 269) and then divides into two afferent renal veins which ascend on the ventral surface of the glands, giving branches to the renal capillary system. About the middle of the kidney each afferent vein is joined by a large transverse branch from the abdominal vein (Fig. 266).

FIG. 266.—Systemic veins of *Iguana tuberculata*. The alimentary canal and appendages, together with the hepatic portal vein and the intrahepatic segment of the postcava, have been removed. The liver occupies the space between the divided ends of the postcava. The vertebral vein represents the rudimentary proximal segment of the postcardinal vein corresponding to the mammalian azygos vein. (Columbia University Museum, No. 1320.)

FIG. 267.—Veins of *Iguana tuberculata*. Connection of systemic veins with sinus venosus of heart. The rudimentary system of the vertebral (azygos) veins and their proximal connection with the subclavian vein are shown. (Columbia University Museum, No. 1859.)

FIG. 268.—Corrosion preparation of venous system of liver in *Iguana tuberculata*. The hepatic portal system and its connection with the abdominal vein, as well as the relation to the postcava, are shown. The preparation supplements Fig. 266, showing the parts which have been removed in the latter. (Columbia University Museum, No. 1860.)

FIG. 269.—*Iguana tuberculata*, ♂. Genito-urinary tract, dorsal view, with renal-portal, postcardinal, and postcaval veins. (Columbia University Museum, No. 1862.)

The renal efferent system begins by a number of inter-renal anastomoses which unite along the mesal border of the right kidney into a large ascending trunk, while the corresponding vessel of the left side, starting from the same anastomosis, is considerably smaller (Figs. 266 and 269). Each of these vessels also receives blood from the testis, epididymis, vas deferens and adrenal body in the male, and from the ovary and oviduct in the female. They represent, in fact, the distal functional part of the right and left embryonic postcardinal vein. Just caudad of the left testis the vein of the left side crosses obliquely ventrad of the aorta and joins the right vessel to form the trunk of the postcava, which enters, immediately beyond the cephalic pole of the right testis, the prolonged caval lobe of the liver (Figs. 266 and 269). Ascending in the substance of this gland and receiving the afferent hepatic veins (Fig. 268), the vena cava emerges from the cephalic surface of the liver greatly enlarged and proceeds to the right auricle.

The abdominal vein divides below into two branches which pass caudad on each side of the bladder, receiving tributaries from the same, to the lateral border of the kidneys (Figs. 266 and 269). Here the vessel is connected by the transverse branch above described with the afferent renal portal system derived from the caudal vein. At the same point it receives the sciatic vein, the principal venous vessel of the posterior extremity. Above, the main abdominal vein, resulting from the union of the two branches referred to, ascends on the dorsal surface of the ventral abdominal wall, receiving a few twigs from the ventral mesogastrium within whose free caudal edge the vessel runs. Just before reaching the liver the abdominal vein turns dorsad on the caudal surface of the gland and joins the hepatic portal vein (Figs. 268 and275). Several accessory veins, two or three in number, belonging to the system of the abdominal vein, pass above this point from the ventral body wall between the layers of the ventral mesogastrium, to enter the liver separately on its convex ventral surface, above the fusion of the main abdominal vein with the portal vein. These additional branches on entering the liver join the portal system, forming a set of ventral accessory portal veins.

The hepatic portal vein derives its principal tributaries from the splenic, gastric, pancreatic and intestinal veins. One or two additional branches (accessory vertebral portal veins), as above stated, connect the system of the segmental and vertebral veins with the portal circulation, entering the liver separately. In like manner one or two gastric veins (accessory gastric portal veins) enter the dorsal aspect of the liver separately, passing from the stomach to the gland between the layers of the gastro-hepatic omentum (Fig. 275).

Compared with the development of the mammalian type, the venous system of Iguana serves to illustrate the stage in the history of the umbilical vein (represented by the abdominal vein of the reptile) in which the connection of the vessel with the portal vein has been formed and transmits the greater part of the blood returned by the umbilical vein to the liver, while the proximal segment above this point, originally continued into the sinus venosus, has begun to disappear, being, however, still represented by the vessels which, as accessory ventral portal veins, pass in the ventral mesogastrium, from the body wall to the liver.

It will be noted that all the hepatic portal blood, whether conducted by the main portal and abdominal vein, or by the accessory portal branches, traverses the capillary circulation of the liver before entering the postcava.

The vertebral and segmental venous system, representing the azygos veins of the mammalia, is very rudimentary (Figs. 266 and 267). The distal portions of the postcardinal veins form the efferent renal branches and the ascending trunks of the postcava.

The next segment of the vertebral veins appears as a trunk on the right side which enters the portal circulation. A second vein higher up is connected with both the gastric portal system and with the longitudinal chain of the vertebral veins. Finally a proximal venous branch on each side of the vertebral column, representing the upper portion of the postcardinal veins, receives the proximal segmental veins and empties into the subclavian vein (Fig. 267).

FIG. 270.—Veins of pigeon, *Columba livia*. (Modified from Parker and Haswell.) The renal-portal vein of the right side is supposed to be dissected to show its passage through the right kidney.

4. Bird.—The characteristic change in the venous system of the bird, as compared with that of the amphibian and reptile, is found in the nearly complete abolition of the renal portal system. The caudal vein bifurcates, sending on each side a large trunk, which receives the pelvic (int. iliac) veins, to the kidney (renal afferent portal vein), but only a few small branches enter the substance of the gland (Fig. 270, afferent renal V). The main vessel continues cephalad through the kidney and, after receiving the vein from the posterior extremity (femoral), unites as common iliac vein with the vessel of the opposite side to form the postcava. This vessel traverses the liver, receiving the hepatic afferent veins of the portal system. The portal vein is formed by tributaries from the intestinal canal, pancreas and spleen, and is also joined by a large coccygeo-mesenteric vein, which is given off at the point of bifurcation of the caudal vein and receives tributaries from the lower part of the alimentary canal. The abdominal vein of amphibians and reptiles is represented probably by the epigastric vein, which returns the blood from the omental mass of fat to the hepatic veins.

Compared with the mammal on the one hand, and with the lower types on the other, the venous circulation of the bird illustrates the following points:

1. Extensive reduction of the renal portal system and direct formation of postcava by the iliac veins, foreshadowing the condition found in the mammal.

2. Complete separation of the portal and systemic venous circulation in the adult. Disappearance of the ventral abdominal vein as a vessel of the body wall.

5. Human Fœtus at Term.—The student is recommended to examine, by dissection and injection, the venous system of a fœtus at term, noting the following facts:

FIG. 271.—Human fœtus at term. Corrosion preparation of heart and vascular system. (Columbia University Museum, No. 1858.)

1. Course of umbilical vein in ventral abdominal wall and along free edge of falciform ligament to liver (Fig. 241), corresponding to the position of the amphibian and reptilian abdominal vein (Figs. 264 and275).

2. Connection of umbilical vein in liver:
(*a*) With portal system (Figs. 258 and 271).
(α) With portal vein.
(β) With portal system of left and quadrate lobes by branches derived directly from umbilical vein while situated in the umbilical fissure (Fig. 258).
(*b*) With hepatic veins and postcava by the ductus venosus (Figs. 258 and 271).

3. Connection of the postcaval and precaval systems by the azygos veins representing the proximal segments of the embryonic postcardinal veins (Fig. 272).

FIG. 272.—Human fœtus at term. Postcava and azygos veins. (Columbia University Museum, No. 1861.)

If possible the dissection of an injected fœtus should be combined with the examination of corrosion preparation of the fœtal circulation and especially of the venous system of the fœtal liver (Figs. 258 and 271).

3. The remnants of fœtal structures in the adult liver (round ligament and ligament of the ductus venosus) should be compared with the structures from which they are derived in the fœtus at term (umbilical vein and ductus venosus).

II. THE VENTRAL MESOGASTRIUM.

This membrane has been heretofore mentioned on several occasions. It now remains for us to carefully consider its arrangement in detail, both as regards the peritoneal relations of the liver and in reference to its influence on the abdominal space as a whole. We can best accomplish this purpose by considering the membrane in the first place in a purely schematic manner. In contradistinction to the primitive common dorsal mesentery, which extends the entire length of the alimentary tube, the ventral mesentery, or properly the ventral mesogastrium, is confined to the stomach and proximal portion of the duodenum. We can represent the membrane as extending between the ventral abdominal wall and the ventral border (later the lesser curvature) of the stomach and of the hepatic angle of the duodenum. Cephalad it is connected with the embryonic septum transversum (future diaphragm). Caudad its two layers pass into each other in a free concave edge, including between them the umbilical vein (free edge of falciform ligament of adult). Consequently a schematic profile or lateral view of the membrane and its attachments in the earlier stages would appear as represented in Fig. 273, while the arrangement in transection would be as shown in Fig. 274. It will be observed that the separation of the cephalic portion of the abdominal cavity into symmetrical right and left halves, previously indicated in discussing the primitive stomach and the dorsal mesogastrium, is actually completed by the ventral mesogastrium. This complete separation of the lateral halves of the cœlom cavity ceases at the point where the ventral mesogastrium terminates in the free concave edge carrying the umbilical vein. Hence caudad of this falciform edge the two halves of the cavity communicate freely with each other ventrad of the intestine and dorsal mesentery.

FIG. 273.—Schematic profile view of ventral mesogastrium with developing liver.

FIG. 274.—Schematic transection of abdomen in region of ventral mesogastrium.

This difference in the extent of the mesogastria is perhaps best understood by reference to their relation to the first portion of the duodenum. We have seen that the duodenum in the early stages is attached dorsally by a portion of the common dorsal mesentery, which, after differentiation of the intestinal tract, immediately follows the dorsal

81

mesogastrium proper, forming the mesoduodenum (Fig. 172). The proximal portion of the duodenum (hepatic angle) is still included within the fold of the ventral mesogastrium which membrane terminates immediately beyond this point in the free edge surrounding the umbilical vein (subsequent round ligament) (Fig. 172). The remainder of the duodenum is devoid of any ventral attachment, being only connected to the dorsal body wall by the mesoduodenum (Fig. 197).

Subsequently, after the fourth month, while the right surface of the mesoduodenum and descending duodenum adhere to the parietal peritoneum, the peritoneal investment of the first portion or hepatic angle remains free. This peritoneal covering of the proximal duodenal segment is situated at the point where the caudal end of the ventral mesogastrium, after surrounding the first portion of the duodenum, becomes continuous with the dorsal mesentery forming the mesoduodenum. Obliteration of the latter membrane by adhesion to the parietal peritoneum leaves the first portion of the duodenum invested on both surfaces by the *lesser omentum*, derived from the ventral mesogastrium. The ventral surface of the gut is covered by the ventral layer, the dorsal surface by the dorsal layer of the lesser omentum. These two layers become continuous around the right free edge of the lesser omentum (hepato-duodenal ligament) forming the ventral boundary of the foramen of Winslow (cf. infra, p. 177).

Returning to the schematic consideration of the ventral mesogastrium above outlined (Figs. 273 and 274) we have to note the first important change in the arrangement depending upon the development of the liver. This organ, growing, as we have seen, from the duodenum, extends between the two layers of the ventral mesogastrium, receiving a serous investment from the same. At an early period the liver, developing thus between the mesogastric layers, reaches the septum transversum and becomes closely connected with it, laying the foundation for the subsequent extensive attachment of the gland to the diaphragm.

Extending caudad the liver grows beyond the caudal free edge of the ventral mesogastrium on each side, carrying the serosa with it. Consequently the ventral margin of the liver becomes indented at this point; the umbilical vein and subsequently its fibrous remnant, the round ligament, are imbedded in a notch and fissure (umbilical notch and fissure) continued from the ventral margin dorsad along the caudal surface of the liver (Fig. 259).

This growth of the liver has now effected a division of the primitive ventral mesogastrium into two segments:

1. Ventral portion, between diaphragm and liver, forms the broad falciform or suspensory ligament of the liver.

2. The dorsal portion, between liver and stomach, forms the lesser or gastro-hepatic omentum.

The caudal free edge of the ventral mesogastrium extends between the umbilicus and the caudal surface of the liver, carrying the umbilical vein between its layers. The growth of the liver serves to bury this free edge and the contained vein in a fissure on the caudal surface of the liver. The same obtains in the case of the ductus venosus continued from the umbilical vein (umbilical fissure and fissure of ductus venosus of adult liver). Consequently the original continuity of the broad ligament and lesser omentum, as parts of the primitive ventral mesogastrium, is not readily seen in the adult.

The broad ligament extends across the convex cephalic surface of the liver uniting it to the ventral abdominal wall and diaphragm, while its free falciform edge apparently stops at the umbilical notch in the ventral border of the organ. Actually, however, the obliterated vein is surrounded in the bottom of the fissure, by a peritoneal fold which effects the junction between broad ligament and lesser omentum.

We will see later in what way the permanent adult arrangement of the lesser omentum is brought about. For the present we can state, on the hand of the schematic Fig. 273, that the free caudal edge of the falciform ligament containing the umbilical vein, and the free edge of the gastro-hepatic omentum form together originally the caudal free edge of the ventral mesogastrium, which membrane becomes separated, by the growth of the liver, into suspensory or broad ligament and lesser or gastro-hepatic omentum.

FIG. 275.—Abdominal viscera of *Iguana tuberculata*. (Columbia University Museum, No. 1313.)

This primitive disposition of the ventral mesogastrium and the viscera connected with the same, is well shown in some of the lower vertebrates in whom the development never proceeds beyond the early mammalian stages. Fig. 275 shows in profile view from the right side the situs viscerum and peritoneum in *Iguana tuberculata*.[5] The two dorsal aortic roots are seen to unite to form the main aorta, which descends between the layers of the dorsal mesentery, sending branches to the dorsal margin of œsophagus and stomach. From the opposite border of the stomach the ventral mesogastrium is derived. Its dorsal segment (gastro-hepatic omentum) connects liver and stomach, carrying between its layers the portal vessels, hepatic artery and biliary duct. The ventral segment of the membrane, forming the suspensory or broad ligament, extends between abdominal wall and ventral surface of the liver. Caudad, the lesser omentum and the suspensory ligament are seen to have a common concave falciform edge.

The ventral abdominal vein ascends between the layers of the suspensory ligament and near the liver becomes connected by a large branch with the portal vein. A few smaller branches are seen passing from the abdominal wall beyond this point. In this reptile, therefore, the permanent vascular arrangement corresponds to an early human embryonic stage.

The reptilian ventral abdominal vein is the homologue of the umbilical vein of the placentalia. The large branch passing to the portal vein represents the connection established in the human embryo between the umbilical and portal veins. The small branches, continuing cephalad between the mesogastric layers, represent the temporary proximal remnants which in the human embryo the umbilical veins form in connection with abdominal walls. The permanent adult arrangement of this part of the vascular system in this animal corresponds therefore to one of the stages of development in the human embryo, as previously indicated (cf. p. 149; Figs. 251 and 252).

PERITONEAL RELATIONS OF LIVER.

It is well to begin the study of the peritoneal connections of the liver with the consideration of the embryonic stage shown in Fig. 273 schematically.

FIG. 276.—Schematic view of embryonic liver detached from its connections, seen from behind, with lines of peritoneal reflection.

If we imagine this embryonic liver detached from its connections in such a manner as to leave the divided peritoneal layers of the ventral mesogastrium as long as possible, and if we regard the preparation from behind, the appearance of the parts could be represented in Fig. 276.[6]

It will of course be seen that the area of direct adhesion to the diaphragm, extending transversely, would separate the lesser omentum from the suspensory ligament.

As is seen in the transection (Fig. 274), the right and left layers of the suspensory ligament, at its attachment to the liver, turn into the visceral peritoneum investing the organ on its ventral and cephalic surfaces. Continuing around the borders of the liver this visceral peritoneum then invests in like manner the dorsal or caudal surface directed toward the stomach, until, at the region of the future portal or transverse fissure, this visceral peritoneum becomes in turn continuous with the two layers of the lesser or gastro-hepatic omentum. Consequently in the embryonic detached liver the lines of peritoneal reflection would be nearly cruciform, the vertical limb of the cross being formed on the cephalic surface by the two layers of the suspensory ligament, while on the caudal surface it is formed by the layers of the lesser omentum. The horizontal arm of the cross is formed by the upper and lower limits of the area of diaphragmatic attachment, along which the parietal diaphragmatic peritoneum turns into the visceral hepatic investment (forming the two layers of the primitive coronary ligament). In the liver shown thus schematically from behind we would overlook the dorsal and adjoining portions of the cephalic and caudal surfaces of the adult human liver.

The primitive biliary duct, portal vein and hepatic artery reach the liver between the layers of the lesser omentum. The venæ revehentes (hepatic veins) reach the sinus venosus at the attachment of the liver to the septum transversum (primitive diaphragm).

83

The first important change, resulting in a rearrangement of these peritoneal layers, is produced by the connection of the umbilical with the rudimentary portal vein.

FIG. 277.—Schematic view of embryonic liver, showing influence of vascular connections on the arrangement of the lines of peritoneal reflection.

FIG. 278.—Later stages, showing development of transverse fissure, Spigelian and caudate lobes.

This junction occupies a relatively wide area on the caudal surface of the liver, and the layers of the lesser omentum are separated somewhat at this point to accommodate the enlarging vascular structures between them. More especially is this the case with the right leaf of the primitive gastro-hepatic omentum. A species of lateral diverticulum is formed by this leaf so as to include the umbilical vein at its junction with the portal. The membrane in the region of this diverticulum turns its surfaces dorsad and ventrad, and its free edge toward the right (Fig. 277). With the gradual increase in the size of the vessels, and with thetransverse position which the rotation of the stomach imparts to the opposite border of the lesser omentum attached to the lesser curvature, this transversely disposed portion gradually exceeds in length and size the part of the original omentum enclosing the umbilical vein. This vessel and the investing peritoneum become lodged in a sagittal depression on the caudal surface of the liver (rudimentary umbilical fissure), while the transverse portion, developed as indicated, surrounds the structures connected with the liver at the future transverse or portal fissure.

Schematically this rearrangement of the hepatic peritoneal lines of reflection can be shown in Fig. 278.

It will be observed that in this way a small part of the caudal surface of the right lobe has become partially marked off from the remainder as a rudimentary Spigelian lobe, bounded ventrally by the transverse fissure and lesser omentum attached to the same; to the left by the two layers of the lesser omentum containing the ductus venosus; while the limit cephalad is afforded by the reflection of peritoneum from liver to diaphragm, forming part of caudal layer of right coronary ligament. To the right this rudimentary Spigelian surface is directly continuous with the rest of the dorsal and caudal surface of the right lobe (Fig. 277). Finally a definite right limit is given to the Spigelian lobe by the increasing size of the postcava and its closer connection with the liver. This vessel now assumes the position of the main venous trunk entering the heart from below.

This inclusion of the vena cava in the fissure or fossa of that name on the dorsal surface of the liver affords, so to speak, the vertical measure of the non-peritoneal area of the liver attached directly to the diaphragm. As the vein develops the interval between the two layers of the right coronary ligament increases, producing the well-known large non-peritoneal area on the dorsal surface of the adult liver, which is directly attached to the diaphragm.

Immediately to the left of the vena cava, however, the original condition persists. The area of direct diaphragmatic attachment is narrow and consequently the two layers of the coronary ligament are close together at this point.[7]

In this way a species of recess (Spigelian recess or hepatic antrum of lesser sac) is formed. A portion of the dorsal liver surface lying just to the left of the vena cava, between it and the ductus venosus, remains invested by peritoneum which is reflected from the boundaries of this space to the diaphragm. This forms the Spigelian lobe (Fig. 278).

The lobe is bounded to the right by the postcava, to the left by the reflection of the lesser omentum to the stomach along the fissure for the ductus venosus; cephalad the boundary is formed by the reflection of the caudal layer of the coronary ligament to the diaphragm.

The caudal boundary is afforded by the transverse position which the lesser omentum has assumed in the region of the transverse or portal fissure.

It will be seen that the original continuity of the Spigelian lobe with the caudal surface of the right lobe is maintained by the narrow bridge of liver tissue connecting the caudal right angle of the rectangular Spigelian lobe with the right lobe. This narrow isthmus, situated between vena cava dorsad and the free right edge of lesser omentum ventrad, forms the so-called *caudate lobe.*

FIG. 279.—Liver of human fœtus at eighth month. View of caudal and dorsal surfaces. (Columbia University Museum, No. 1854.)

FIG. 280.—Human fœtal liver at term, showing lines of peritoneal reflection on cephalic, dorsal, and caudal surfaces. (Columbia University Museum, No. 1855.)

Fig. 279 shows a human fœtal liver at the end of the eighth month in the view from below and behind. The original continuity of the layers of the lesser omentum, attached along the fissure for the ductus venosus, with the fold of the falciform ligament occupying the umbilical fissure can still be made out for a short distance beyond the left extremity of the transverse fissure. The section of the lesser omentum which occupies the transverse fissure and, including the portal vein, hepatic artery and duct between its layers, terminates in the free right margin, is evidently derived by a lateral extension from the right layer of the primitive sagittal lesser omentum, whose original direction is preserved along the fissure of the ductus venosus.

In Fig. 280 the lines of peritoneal reflection on the cephalic, dorsal and caudal surfaces of a human fœtal liver at term are shown.

We can now proceed to trace the reflection of the peritoneum from the liver to adjacent structures.

Begin with the caudal layer of the coronary ligament on the extreme right, where fusion with the corresponding cephalic layer produces the right triangular ligament. The caudal layer of the coronary ligament proceeds from right to left along the caudal margin of the non-peritoneal dorsal diaphragmatic surface of right lobe, being reflected along this line from the liver to the adjacent portions of the diaphragm and ventral surface of right kidney and suprarenal capsule (hepato-renal ligament). A small cephalic part of ventral surface of right suprarenal capsule lies above this line of reflection, is hence non-peritoneal and firmly connected with the liver just to the left of entrance of vena cava into the caval fissure. Continuing, the caudal layer of the coronary ligament crosses the ventral surface of the vena cava and turns, immediately to the left of the vein, at a right angle, ascending to form the left boundary of the Spigelian recess, being reflected along this line from the left margin of the caval fissure to the pillars of the diaphragm. Arrived at the opening of the central tendon permitting passage of vena cava into pericardium, and at the level of the entrance of the left hepatic vein into the cava, the peritoneum turns again at a right angle and runs from right to left, forming the cephalic limit of the Spigelian recess. Turning caudad along the fissure for the ductus venosus, as right leaf of that portion of the lesser omentum which is attached to this fissure and has preserved its sagittal position, the peritoneal line of reflection reaches the left extremity of the portal or transverse fissure. It now turns to the right following the fissure as the dorsal layer of the transverse segment of the lesser omentum, and becomes continuous, with the formation of a free right edge, with the ventral layer of the same membrane, passing from right to left, the two layers including between them the structures entering and leaving the liver at the transverse fissure (portal vein, hepatic artery, duct). Arriving at the left extremity of the transverse fissure the ventral layer of the transverse segment of the lesser omentum—as we practically trace it in the adult as a free membrane—turns directly into the left leaf of the sagittal segment attached along the fissure for the ductus venosus, and becomes continuous along the dorsal border of the left lobe with the caudal layer of the left coronary ligament. This direct continuity, as just stated, exists practically in the adult. From the development of the membrane, however, it will be seen that the ventral layer of the transverse lesser omentum, at the left extremity of the portal fissure, becomes continuous with the right layer of the primitive mesogastrium enclosing the umbilical vein. After surrounding this vein it is continued into the left leaf of the same membrane, which in turn passes into the left layer of the portion attached along the fissure for the ductus venosus.

This original connection can at times be traced very clearly in young specimens (Fig. 279), and occasionally is also still evident in the adult liver.

85

Usually, however, the round ligament of the adult and its investing peritoneum is buried so deeply in the umbilical fissure, or even bridged over in part by liver tissue, that the connection is not evident. The ventral layer of the transverse omentum then appears directly continuous with the left layer of the sagittal omentum attached along the fissure for the ductus venosus.

We can sum up the facts just considered as follows:

1. The rotation of the stomach from the sagittal into the transverse position, and the development of the umbilical and portal veins, rearrange the original sagittal plane of the lesser omentum, dividing it into two districts:

(*a*) Cephalic portion, remaining in the original sagittal plane, follows the fissure for the ductus venosus. With the incorporation of the Spigelian lobe in the adult dorsal or "posterior" surface of the liver, this segment of the omentum assumes a vertical direction, forming the left boundary of the Spigelian recess, being reflected from the fissure for the ductus venosus to the abdominal portion of the œsophagus and the part of the lesser curvature of stomach adjacent to the cardia.

(*b*) Distal caudal portion of the lesser omentum is twisted laterally and turned to the right by the change in the position of the stomach and the development of the structures connected with the liver at the transverse fissure. It is reflected from this fissure to the distal part of the lesser curvature and to the first portion of the duodenum. This transverse segment of the lesser omentum is a secondary derivative from the right leaf of the primitive membrane, produced by the enlarged area for entrance of umbilical and portal veins at the transverse fissure. It lies ventrad of caudal border of Spigelian lobe.

2. The distal segment of the original omentum containing the umbilical vein (round ligament), continues imbedded in the umbilical fissure, to the ventral margin of the liver, where it joins the layers of the suspensory ligament passing over the cephalic surface.

3. The adult lesser omentum at the transverse fissure may be regarded as a diverticulum of the right leaf of the primitive embryonal sagittal omentum.

With the reduction of the umbilical vein after birth to form the round ligament this structure becomes deeply buried in the umbilical fissure. The ventral and dorsal layers of the lesser omentum at the transverse fissure thus become continuous with respectively the left and right layers of the second segment of the omentum which ascends vertically along the fissure for the ductus venosus.

4. The cephalic layer of the coronary ligament (Fig. 280) remains practically in the embryonic condition. The adult convex cephalic surface of the liver is traversed in the sagittal direction by the suspensory ligament which connects it with the abdominal surface of the diaphragm, and thus effects the division into right and left lobes on the convex surface. Arrived at the dorsal border of this surface (junction of "superior" and "posterior" surfaces) the right and left leaves of the falciform ligament turn at right angles into the cephalic layer of the right and left coronary ligament, which at each extremity meet the right and left caudal layers to form the triangular ligaments. It will thus be seen that the apparent irregularity in the relative arrangement of the s. c. "upper" and "lower" layers of the coronary ligaments, produced by the Spigelian recess, is only a difference in the interval between the two layers, caused by the vertical extent of the non-peritoneal direct diaphragmatic attachment of the right lobe to the right of the vena cava.

Comparative Anatomy of Spigelian Lobe and Vena Cava in the Cat.—The lines of peritoneal reflection in the *cat's* liver and the arrangement of the Spigelian lobe and recess are seen in Fig. 281, taken from a preparation hardened in situ.

FIG. 281.—Liver of cat, hardened *in situ.* (Columbia University Museum, No. 1836.)

FIG. 282.—Dorsal view of human liver and stomach in fœtus at term, showing lines of hepatic and gastric attachment of lesser omentum.

Compared with the human liver it will be noted that the area of diaphragmatic adhesion is much less developed. The dorsal surface of the right lobe to the right of the postcava is peritoneal, there being no extension laterad of the right coronary and triangular ligaments. The postcava enters the liver in a special prolongation of the liver substance (caval lobe).

The boundaries of the Spigelian recess and the lines of attachment of the gastro-hepatic omentum correspond to the human arrangement.

RELATION OF THE HEPATIC PERITONEUM TO THE "LESSER SAC."

Foramen of Winslow.—We have previously seen that the rotation of the stomach and the further growth of the dorsal mesogastrium lead, in the first instance, to the formation of the "lesser peritoneal cavity." This cavity is in fact primarily the retrogastric space created by the transverse position of the stomach, augmented by the cavity of the omental bursa developed from the dorsal mesogastrium.

We have now to consider the additional boundaries of this space contributed by the peritoneal connection of the lesser curvature with the liver.

FIG. 283.—Schema of lines of reflection of peritoneum on dorsal surface of liver and in the formation of the gastro-hepatic omentum. *A B*, transverse section of lesser omentum attached to transverse fissure of liver and to pyloric section of lesser curvature (*A' B'*); *B C*, vertical section of lesser omentum passing between fissure of ductus venosus and cardiac section of lesser curvature of stomach (*B' C'*); *C D*, line of reflection of peritoneum from cephalic border of Spigelian lobe to diaphragm; *D E*, line of reflection of peritoneum from right border of Spigelian lobe to left margin of postcava and diaphragm.

FIG. 284.—Portion of abdominal viscera of adult human subject, hardened *in situ*. (Columbia University, Study Collection.) The segment of stomach between cardiac and pyloric orifices has been removed, dividing the lesser omentum to this extent, but leaving the right extremity of the membrane (lig. hepato-duodenale) intact. Behind this portion the arrow passes through the foramen of Winslow.

FIG. 285.—Liver and stomach of *Macacus pileatus*. (Columbia University, Study Collection.)

FIG. 286.—Abdominal viscera of adult human subject, hardened *in situ*; with liver lifted up after incision of the gastro-hepatic omentum. (Columbia University Museum, No. 1845.)

The lesser omentum follows, of course, along its gastric attachment to the lesser curvature the general direction of the stomach, passing from the cardia transversely downwards and to the right. We distinguish the two layers of the adult membrane as ventral and dorsal, which meet in the free right edge and include between them the main structures entering and leaving the liver at the transverse fissure, viz.: the portal vein, hepatic artery and bile-duct.

The lesser omentum therefore prolongs the plane of the stomach cephalad towards the liver and thus forms the continuation of the ventral boundary of the lesser peritoneal sac. We can now consider the line of its hepatic attachment in the light of the facts previously adduced, and combine the same with the line of gastric attachment to the lesser curvature. Fig. 282 shows the fœtal liver and stomach in their relative position in the dorsal view, and Fig. 283 gives the lines of the peritoneal reflections. The vertical segment of the omentum, occupying the fissure for the ductus venosus, passes to the cardiac part of the lesser curvature, its ventral layer covering the ventral and left side of the œsophagus, while its dorsal layer passes to the dorsal and right side of the œsophagus at its entrance into the stomach. The transverse segment of the omentum, attached on the liver to the portal or transverse fissure, accedes to the pyloric part of the lesser curvature. Of course the ventral and dorsal layers of the omentum are continuous with the serous visceral investment of the ventral and dorsal surfaces of the stomach.

Fig. 284 shows this right-angled course of the lesser omentum at the hepatic line of attachment in a preparation of the abdominal viscera hardened in situ, with the segment of the stomach between the cardiac and pyloric orifices removed. The arrow is passed behind the right free edge of the lesser omentum. This portion of the membrane is still intact, not having been disturbed by the removal of the body of the stomach, and includes between its layers the structures connected with the liver at the transverse fissure (duct, hepatic artery and portal vein). The lesser omentum is seen to be attached to the liver along the transverse

87

fissure (Fig. 284, *A*) and along the fissure for the ductus venosus (Fig. 284, *B*), constituting the transverse and vertical segments above referred to, which pass into each other at the angle of junction between the transverse fissure (left end) and the fissure for the ductus venosus (Fig. 284, *C*). The caudal and left border of the Spigelian lobe is exposed by the division of the omentum, and the extent of the Spigelian or hepatic recess of the lesser peritoneal sac is shown. Fig. 285 shows the liver, stomach and lesser omentum of a Macaque monkey hardened in situ, and demonstrates still more conclusively that the uniform curve of the omentum along the lesser curvature of the stomach becomes a broken line at the hepatic attachment, the angle being placed at the left end of the transverse fissure at the point where the same encounters the fissure for the ductus venosus.

In Fig. 286 finally the hardened abdominal viscera of an adult human subject are shown in the ventral view with the lesser omentum incised. The cut through the lesser omentum exposes the hepatic recess of the lesser peritoneal cavity immediately to the left of the foramen of Winslow. Toward the right free margin of the omentum the divided portal vein, hepatic artery and duct are seen between the layers of the omentum imbedded in the pancreas and coursing behind the first portion of the duodenum on their way to the transverse fissure.

To the left of these structures the omental tuberosity of the pancreas projects above the level of the lesser curvature under cover of the secondary parietal peritoneum forming the dorsal wall of the lesser sac, while the lower edge of the Spigelian lobe appears in the upper angle of the incision.

If we remember that the liver is itself welded to the diaphragm between the layers of the coronary ligament (Fig. 280), it will become apparent that the serous surface of the Spigelian lobe forms part of the ventral wall of a peritoneal recess situated behind the lesser omentum, between this membrane and the diaphragm. Access to this recess, without the division of peritoneal layers, can only be obtained by passing from right to left, along the caudate lobe, between the vena cava behind, covered by parietal peritoneum, and the free right edge of the lesser omentum in front. (In the reverse direction of the arrow shown inFig. 284.) This hepatic or Spigelian recess of the lesser peritoneal cavity has categorically the following boundaries (Figs. 282 and 283):

Dorsal: Parietal peritoneum, reflected along the line CD, from the caudal layer of the coronary ligament to the diaphragm.

Ventral: Visceral peritoneum investing the Spigelian lobe and the gastro-hepatic omentum.

Right: Reflection of peritoneum along the line DE (caval fissure) to become the parietal peritoneum covering the diaphragm.

Left: Right layer of lesser omentum, reflected along the fissure for the ductus venosus (CB) to the cardiac portion of the lesser curvature, continuous with the dorsal layer of the lesser omentum reflected from the transverse fissure to the pyloric segment of the lesser curvature (AB).

We will presently see that certain relations of the vessels connected with the liver at the transverse fissure and of the duodenum prevent the finger, when passed from right to left behind the free right edge of the lesser omentum and along the caudate lobe of the liver, from proceeding downward at this point. A narrow channel of communication is thus formed between the Spigelian recess and rest of the lesser sac on the one hand, and the general greater peritoneal cavity on the other. This channel is the so-called foramen of Winslow.

Having once passed this narrow space the finger will be in the Spigelian recess and can palpate its boundaries. Further progress cephalad and to the right is barred by the diaphragmatic adhesions of the liver just detailed. But in the direction downward behind the lesser omentum and along the dorsal surface of the stomach, as well as to the left toward the spleen the excursion is limited only by the length of the examining finger.

After opening the abdominal cavity of the human adult, elevating the liver and depressing the stomach, the hepatic attachment of the lesser omentum can be traced as already described. It will then be observed that the gastric attachment of the membrane lies in one plane following the lesser curvature while the hepatic attachment forms a broken line, with the angle situated at the left extremity of the transverse fissure. The vertical segment of the hepatic attachment, occupying the fissure for the ductus venosus, turns at this angle into the transverse segment which follows the transverse fissure to its right extremity where the two layers pass into each other around the right free omental margin (hepato-duodenal ligament). Consequently we overlook, in an abdominal cavity thus exposed, the entire caudal surface of the liver, including the caudal surfaces of right, left, and quadrate lobes. The junction of right and caudate lobes can be seen between vena cava and right edge of the omentum, or rather, it can be felt at this point. But the Spigelian lobe, turning its surface dorsad against the parietal peritoneum covering the diaphragm, forms part of the "posterior" liver surface and is not visible, although—as just stated, it can be palpated by passing the finger through the foramen of Winslow. The Spigelian lobe cannot be overlooked in its entire extent until the liver is removed from the body and regarded from behind. The caudal edge (continuation of its right angle into the caudate lobe and papillary tubercle) can be seen by tearing through the layers of the lesser omentum and lifting the liver up forcibly (Fig. 286).

Caudal Boundary of Foramen of Winslow.—We have above referred to the fact that the finger introduced through the foramen of Winslow meets in this canal with resistance if an attempt is made to pass downwards. After passing this constricting point the free excursion into the Spigelian recess and behind the omentum and stomach and toward the spleen can be performed.

In considering the elements which produce this narrowing of the communication between the two peritoneal sacs at the foramen of Winslow we have to deal with two factors, one primary and constant, the other secondary and inconstant.

1. The first of these is afforded by the arrangement of the arterial vessel supplying the liver. The hepatic artery is a branch of the cœliac axis, furnishing arterial blood to the liver tissues and supplying, in addition, branches to the stomach, duodenum and pancreas.

This vessel is, of course, placed primarily, like all other arterial branches supplying the alimentary tract, between the layers of the primitive dorsal mesentery. Originally the vessel supplies the distal (pyloric) portion of the stomach along its dorsal attached border (subsequently the greater curvature) corresponding to the adult gastro-epiploica dextra of the hepatic (gastro-duodenalis).

It likewise gives branches to the adjacent pyloric portion of the duodenum and the pancreas, as that gland develops from the intestine, corresponding to the adult superior pancreatico-duodenal branch, and to the ventral border (lesser curvature) of stomach, corresponding to the adult pyloric branch of the hepatic.

With the development of the liver from the duodenum arterial branches derived from this primitive gastro-duodenal vessel pass to the sprouting hepatic cylinders by continuing around the duodenum, beneath its serous investment, to reach the interval between the two layers of the ventral mesogastrium, in which the liver develops, near the free margin of this membrane.

After the rotation, which turns the right side of the stomach, duodenum and mesoduodenum dorsad, the branch which passes over the dorsal surface of the duodenum to reach the liver becomes more favorably situated and develops into the main hepatic artery which reaches the liver at the transverse fissure between the folds of the lesser omentum. The original right side of the duodenum, now turned dorsad, adheres to the parietal peritoneum. The hepatic artery which reached the liver by passing over this surface of the duodenum, beneath its visceral serous covering, becomes imbedded in connective tissue by the adhesion of the visceral duodenal and the primitive parietal peritoneum. Hence in the adult the hepatic artery courses imbedded in the connective tissue which binds the duodenum to the abdominal background to reach the interval between the two omental layers which carry it to the transverse fissure.

The hepatic artery, therefore, derived from one of the primitive intestinal branches (gastro-duodenal) is, notwithstanding its hidden position in the adult, originally situated between the layers of the free primitive dorsal mesogastrium.

FIG. 287.—Primitive dorsal and ventral mesogastrium with course of hepatic artery.

It now becomes necessary to regard the development of the great omentum from the primitive dorsal mesogastrium in relation to this course of the hepatic artery. We have seen that the great omentum and the cavity of the omental bursa is produced by the extension of the dorsal mesogastrium to the left and caudad, subsequent to the rotation of the stomach. The splenic artery and the left gastro-epiploic branch pass from the cœliac axis to the left between the layers of the mesogastrium, as previously seen (Figs. 291 and 292).

The hepatic artery, however, is so to speak placed on the border line between the portion of the primitive mesentery which, as dorsal mesogastrium, is to turn to the left and caudad to form the great omentum, and the portion which, as mesoduodenum, turns to the right and passes to the duodenal loop (Fig. 287).

In the further course of development the dorsal mesogastrium grows more and more, forming the omental bag, while the mesoduodenum on the other hand becomes anchored early and obliterated as a free membrane by adhesion of its original right layer to the primitive parietal peritoneum. The hepatic artery runs on the line dividing these two different mesenteric segments. We can imagine, so to speak, that the redundant growth of the omentum to the left and caudad, takes place over the hepatic artery as a resistant support (Figs. 288 and 289). Cephalad of the hepatic artery is the developing omentum, caudad of the vessel the mesoduodenum. The artery follows the cephalic limit of the mesoduodenum and becomes, as stated, adherent to the abdominal background in the segment between its origin from the cœliac axis and the point where, after having crossed the dorsal surface of the duodenum, it enters the right edge of the lesser omentum on its way to the liver.

FIG. 288.—The liver divides the ventral mesogastrium into a dorsal segment, the gastro-hepatic or lesser omentum, and a ventral segment, the suspensory or falciform ligament of the liver.

FIG. 289.—Stages in the development of the dorsal mesogastrium (omental bursa) and mesoduodenum to show relation of hepatic artery to these two segments of the primitive common dorsal mesentery.

Pancreatico-gastric Folds.—If we open the lesser peritoneal cavity by dividing the gastro-hepatic omentum and look into the background of the retro-omental space, we will see a fold of the secondary lining parietal peritoneum (derived from the mesogastrium), which can be traced from the cephalic border of the pancreas to the pyloric extremity of the stomach. This fold carries the hepatic artery to the lesser omentum behind the first portion of the duodenum, and is called the right or main pancreatico-gastric fold. A similar fold, further to the left, carries in a like manner the coronary artery of the stomach to the cardiac end of the lesser curvature. This fold forms the left or secondary pancreatico-gastric fold. Between the two folds the caudal margin of the Spigelian lobe projects into the lesser cavity.

The appearance of the two pancreatico-gastric folds in the adult human subject is well seen in Fig. 284.

FIG. 290.—Abdominal viscera of *Nasua rufa*, brown coaiti, with stomach turned up and great omentum divided. (From a fresh dissection.)

FIG. 291.—Schematic transection through foramen of Winslow before adhesion of dorsal mesogastrium and mesoduodenum to parietal peritoncum.

FIG. 292.—The same section after the adult conditions have been established by adhesion.

Fig. 290 shows the abdominal cavity of*Nasua rufa*, with great omentum divided to bring into view the vessels passing from cœliac axis to liver and stomach and elevating the retrogastric parietal peritoneum to produce the pancreatico-gastric folds.

(The course of the hepatic artery from cœliac axis to liver in the dorsal view in the cat is seen inFig. 223.)

Figs. 291 and 292 represent schematically cross-sections directly through the foramen of Winslow, showing the method by means of which the hepatic artery reaches the upper border of the duodenum and the effect of the adhesion of duodenum and mesoduodenum upon the disposition of the vessel.

The coronary artery, like the splenic, is at first situated between the layers of the dorsal mesogastrium (vertebro-splenic segment). Like the splenic the coronary artery becomes anchored to the abdominal background and placed secondarily behind the parietalperitoneum of the lesser sac by the adhesion of this mesogastric segment to the primitive parietal peritoneum. To reach the lesser curvature at the cardia and to run thence from left to right along the lesser curvature between the layers of the gastro-hepatic omentum, the vessel raises the investing parietal peritoneum (originally the right leaf of the dorsal mesogastrium) into a crescentic fold, extending between its origin from the cœliac axis at cephalic margin of pancreas and the beginning of the lesser curvature of the stomach. Hence this fold is called the left pancreatico-gastric fold. (Seen well in Fig. 284.)

In the next place it must be borne in mind that the relation of the primitive hepatic artery to the vascular supply of the stomach, pancreas and duodenum produces a permanent shortening of the primitive mesentery at this point. This result is indicated in the schematic figures 287, 288 and 289.

In the original condition the dorsal mesentery, passing to a practically straight intestinal tube, is of uniform sagittal measure (Fig. 287).

As development proceeds, and as the liver grows from the duodenum, the hepatic artery develops from the primitive pyloric vessel as above indicated. This vessel, assuming greater importance with the rapid growth of the liver, is not lengthened out as happens with the remaining purely intestinal branches which follow the increase in the length of the intestinal canal. The hepatic artery, therefore, will mark the point where the original short sagittal extent of the primitive mesentery will tend to be preserved. Cephalad of this point the dorsal mesogastrium grows out into the great omentum (Figs. 288 and 289); caudad of the same point the membrane, in following the development of the intestine, becomes drawn out into the permanent mesentery and mesocolon.

The hepatic artery, in addition, marks the cephalic limit of the adhesion which anchors the duodenum and mesoduodenum to the parietal peritoneum. Consequently in the adult the vessel courses in as direct a manner as possible, taking the shortest course from the cœliac axis to the liver, passing dorsad of the duodenum and giving what now appear as secondary branches to supply the intestine, the stomach and pancreas (pyloric and gastro-duodenal arteries (pancreatico-duod. superior and gastro-epiploica dextra)).

Even if no fixation of the duodenum and mesoduodenum takes place this course of the hepatic artery will produce a constricted passage between the liver (caudate lobe) cephalad, abdominal parietes and aorta dorsad, lesser omentum and pyloric duodenum ventrad, and hepatic artery caudad. This passage leading from the general peritoneal cavity into the retrogastric space is the *primitive foramen of Winslow*. This condition is well represented in the abdominal cavity of some of the lower mammalia, in which duodenum and mesoduodenum remain permanently free.

Fig. 293 shows a view of the abdominal cavity from the right side in a specimen of the ant-eater, *Tamandua bivittata*.

FIG. 293.—Abdominal viscera of *Tamandua bivittata*, the little ant-eater, with the intestines turned downward and to the left. (From a fresh dissection.)

FIG. 294.—Schematic sagittal section through foramen of Winslow before fixation of pancreas by adhesion of mesoduodenum.

FIG. 295.—The same section after adhesion of mesoduodenum and pancreas. The pancreas appears secondarily retroperitoneal, after adhesion of apposed surfaces of mesoduodenum and primitive parietal peritoneum over dotted area, producing fixation of dorsal surface of pancreas.

The right kidney is seen in the background, covered by the parietal peritoneum. The duodenum and mesoduodenum are free and can be turned toward the median line. The opening of the foramen of Winslow leading into the retrogastric space is seen between the liver cephalad, kidney and vena cava dorsad, lesser omentum and pyloric extremity of the stomach ventrad, and a fold of peritoneum carrying the hepatic artery caudad. Exactly similar conditions prevail in the cat and in many other mammals.

It will be seen in all these instances that neither portal vein nor bile-ducts limit the foramen caudad. These structures can be lifted up and turned toward the median line with the free duodenum and mesoduodenum. But the hepatic artery must pass to the liver from the *retroperitoneal cœliac axis*. In doing this the vessel traverses the cephalic border of the pancreas, and the pyloric extremity of the stomach and duodenum, to reach the lesser omentum which conveys it to the liver.

Consequently there must always be a narrow peritoneal neck between the liver cephalad, aorta dorsad, hepatic artery caudad, and pyloric extremity of stomach and duodenum together with the lesser omentum ventrad. It should be remembered that the vessel which extends after the development of the liver into the lesser omentum as the *hepatic* artery, was originally destined for the supply of these latter structures. In the adult these primary embryonic terminal branches to the intestine appear as secondary branches derived from the hepatic as the main vessel. Their origin, however, serves to keep the beginning of the small intestine in comparatively close connection with the hepatic artery which courses over the dorsal surface of the duodenum to reach the liver. The narrow space thus left between aorta, hepatic artery, duodenum, lesser omentum and liver forms the framework of the foramen of Winslow and appears always as a confined and narrow channel. This relation is shown in the accompanying schematic Figs. 294 and 295 which represent a sagittal section through the foramen. This primitive foramen is thus bounded cephalad by the liver (caudate lobe, connecting Spigelian and right lobes), ventrad by the first portion of the duodenum and the lesser omentum, with hepatic artery behind the intestine and between the omental layers; dorsad by the abdominal background and large retroperitoneal vessels, and caudad by the cœliac axis and beginning of the hepatic artery.

2. In the forms which possess in the adult an adherent duodenum and mesoduodenum, as in man, the foramen of Winslow obtains a secondary caudal limit by the agglutination of the descending duodenum and the parietal prerenal peritoneum. This is the secondary and inconstant factor referred to above in the caudal boundary of the foramen. The result of this anchoring of duodenum and mesoduodenum is to bring the margin of the foramen further to the right and to bury the hepatic artery still further from view. Thus in the adult human subject the structures bounding the foramen at the margin of the entrance into the narrow channel would be above caudate lobe of liver, behind postcava, below duodenum adherent to ventral surface of right kidney, in front first portion of duodenum and lesser omentum. The hepatic artery will be felt on introducing the finger through the foramen in its original position, but it will be seen that the actual boundaries of the foramen have been moved so to speak a little further to the right by the duodenal adhesion.

FIG. 296.—Dissection of adult liver, pancreas, spleen, and duodenum, with vessels, to show structures concerned in the formation of the foramen of Winslow. (Columbia University, Study Collection.)

Fig. 296 shows a complete dissection of the adult human viscera and vessels concerned in the formation of the foramen, hardened in situ.

The stomach is removed, dividing of course the coronary artery and vein and the left gastro-epiploic artery. The portal vein, hepatic artery and bile-duct are seen entering and leaving the liver at the transverse fissure. Behind them and to the right the vena cava enters the liver. The hepatic artery distributes its pancreatico-duodenal branches to the duodenum and pancreas. The left angle of the Spigelian lobe and the fissure for the ductus venosus appear to the left of the portal vein and hepatic artery. The right angle of the Spigelian lobe and its continuation into the right lobe by means of the caudate lobe is hidden by the structures occupying the transverse fissure. We would enter the beginning of the foramen of Winslow by passing between the vena cava behind, the structures in the transverse fissure (portal vein, hepatic artery and duct) in front, caudate lobe of liver above and duodenum below, the latter in the undisturbed condition of the parts adherent to the right kidney. Continuing to the left the finger would pass between aorta behind, cœliac axis and hepatic artery below and in front, and liver above. These structures bound the permanent and primary narrow channel of communication between the retrogastric or lesser peritoneal space and the general peritoneal cavity, which exists even if a free duodenum and mesoduodenum allow us to lift the intestine away from vena cava and right kidney.

The main facts pertaining to the structure of the lesser peritoneal sac and its connection with the greater peritoneal cavity by means of the foramen of Winslow may be summed up as follows:

FIG. 297.—Schematic sagittal section of the ventral and dorsal mesogastria and epiploic bursa in a human embryo of eight weeks. (Modified from Kollmann.)

FIG. 298.—Transection of human embryo of 3 cm., vertex-coccygeal measure. (Kollmann.)

FIG. 299.—Schematic sagittal section of abdomen to illustrate the intestinal branches of the abdominal aorta. The gastric and hepatic arteries are shown for the sake of convenience as arising together from the cœliac axis (B), hence the left and right gastro-pancreatic folds carrying these vessels appear fused at their beginning, separating the hepatic recess of the lesser peritoneal sac (A) from the cavity of the omental bursa (C).

The mesogastrium as a whole, expanding originally in the sagittal plane in a fan-shaped manner between the vertebral column and the ventral abdominal wall, from the level of the umbilicus to the septum transversum (diaphragm), divides the cephalic part of the abdominal cavity into a symmetrical right and left half.

Figs. 172 and 273represent the membrane as seen in a profile view from the left side. We distinguish the segment dorsad of the stomach as the dorsal mesogastrium, directly continuous with the remaining segments of the common primitive dorsal mesentery, while the portion ventrad of the stomach forms the ventral mesogastrium in which the liver develops. The segment of the ventral mesogastrium between liver and stomach becomes the lesser or gastro-hepatic omentum, while that between liver and ventral abdominal wall forms the falciform or suspensory ligament.

A transection, showing the dorsal and ventral mesogastrium at the level of the fundus of the stomach, is given in Fig. 298. The mesogastria are here seen to be short, while in the schematicFigs. 291 and292 the membrane is, for the sake of distinctness, represented as being of considerable extent.

The ventral mesogastrium surrounding the liver and stomach extends caudad to include the first portion of the duodenum. Beyond this point it terminates in a thickened free edge which includes the umbilical vein. This vein extends from the umbilicus to the transverse fissure of the liver (Fig. 297), lying within the umbilical fissure on the caudal surface of the gland.

At the point where the vein enters the liver the thickened margin of the ventral mesogastrium is continued, as ligamentum hepato-duodenale, to the upper part of the duodenum and forms the ventral boundary of the foramen of Winslow. Between the layers of the mesogastrium which meet in this margin are situated the portal vein, biliary duct and hepatic artery, together with the nerves and lymphatics of the liver.

The mesogastrium originally divided the abdominal cavity between umbilicus and diaphragm into symmetrical right and left halves of equal size and extent. This early symmetrical arrangement becomes disturbed about the seventh week by the rotation of the stomach and the resulting altered course of the mesogastrium, which render the two original equal halves of the abdominal cavity unequal and asymmetrical. The original right half becomes placed behind the stomach and is converted into a blind sac with its opening directed to the right.

The communication of the general abdominal cavity with the retrogastric space by means of this channel is still wide in the embryo, but gradually becomes narrowed in the course of further development to form the foramen of Winslow. This opening is situated between the hepato-duodenal ligament and the parietal peritoneum covering the vena cava. It is constricted from below by the curve of the hepatic artery as this vessel passes from the cœliac axis to reach the liver at the transverse fissure between the layers of the lesser omentum.

The earlier developmental stages of the higher mammalian embryos are in general well illustrated by the permanent adult conditions found in some of the lower vertebrates, in which development does not proceed beyond the primitive condition.

In reptiles, birds and mammals the epiploic bursa is generally formed, while in amphibia the dorsal mesogastrium is very short and connects the stomach directly to the dorsal midline of the abdominal cavity without forming the sac-like extension of the great omentum.

The dorsal mesogastrium with the stomach, and the ventral mesogastrium including the liver between its layers, divides in these animals the cephalic part of the body cavity into two halves, corresponding to the earlier embryonic stages in man and in the higher mammalia.

The foramen of Winslow of the higher forms appears in the lower vertebrates as the wide-open space leading from below into the right half of the cœlom cavity. The dorsal mesogastrium remains short, not forming the pouch-like extension of the great omentum. The stomach retains more or less its primitive vertical position without rotation or elevation of the pyloric extremity, and the intestinal canal is simple, short and comparatively straight.

PART III.
LARGE AND SMALL INTESTINE, ILEO-COLIC JUNCTION AND CÆCUM.

In considering the anatomy of the human cæcum and vermiform appendix many structural conditions are encountered which can only be correctly appreciated in the light of the physiology of the digestive tract. The alimentary canal as a whole affords one of the most striking examples of the adaptation of structure to function. The constant renewal of the tissues of the body by the absorption of nutritive material, the necessary concomitant egestion of undigestible remnants, the variety in the quantity and character of the food habitually taken, all serve to explain why the alimentary canal responds structurally in individual forms so completely to the physiological demands made upon it. This will become especially evident if we extend our observations to include, in addition to man, a review of the corresponding structures in representative types of the lower vertebrates. Moreover the human cæcum and appendix are in part rudimentary structures, representing a portion of the alimentary tract which, in accordance with altered conditions of food supply and nutrition, has lost its original functional significance to the organism and which consequently exhibits the wide range of structural variation which characterizes the majority of rudimentary and vestigial organs.

The vermiform process of man and the higher primates is thus one of several indications given in the structure of the alimentary canal (the character of the dentition is another example) which suggests that at one phylogenetic period the forms composing the order or their immediate ancestors were largely or entirely herbivorous, and hence possessed a more extensively developed cæcal apparatus than their omnivorous descendants of to-day. In approaching, therefore, the study of the human cæcum and appendix we will at once meet with conditions which call for the simultaneous physiological and morphological consideration of the adjacent small and large intestine.

Again many of the structural peculiarities which characterize the human cæcal apparatus can only be correctly valued by comparison with the corresponding parts in the lower vertebrates. Our inquiry will, therefore, most profitably include the following subdivisions of the subject:

I. General review of the functional and structural characters of the vertebrate large and small intestine.

II. Systematic consideration of the ileo-colic junction and the connected structures in the vertebrate series.

III. Phylogeny of the types of vertebrate ileo-colic junction and cæcum, and their probable lines of evolution.

IV. Detailed morphology of the human cæcum and vermiform appendix.

I. GENERAL REVIEW OF THE MORPHOLOGY AND PHYSIOLOGY OF THE VERTEBRATE INTESTINE.

We have seen that the intestinal tube of all vertebrates is the product of two of the embryonal blastodermic layers, the entoderm and mesoderm. The former furnishes the characteristic and cardinal elements of the digestive tract, viz., the secretory and absorbing

94

epithelium of the mucous membrane and of the accessory digestive glands, the liver and pancreas.

From the mesoderm, on the other hand, are derived the muscular and connective tissue coats which surround the epithelial tube and contribute to the thickness of the intestinal wall, as well as the blood vessels and lymphatics. The alimentary canal separates from the yolk-sac of the embryo by the development of cranial, caudal and lateral folds, and at an early period communicates with the neural canal by the primitive postanal gut (cf. p. 23). This connection subsequently becomes lost. The oral and anal openings, by means of which the alimentary canal communicates with the exterior, are formed *secondarily* by entodermal invaginations which finally break through into the lumen of the canal (cf. p. 24).

At an early embryonic stage the alimentary canal appears therefore as a straight cylindrical tube running cephalo-caudad in the long axis of the body-cavity, and suspended by the primitive mesentery from the ventral aspect of the chorda dorsalis.

In Amphioxus, the cyclostomata, certain teleosts, dipnœans and lower amphibians the canal remains permanently in this condition (cf. Fig. 310).

In the remaining vertebrates the uniform non-differentiated tube of the embryo develops further and appears more or less distinctly divided into a proximal segment, the *foregut*, a central segment, the *midgut*, and a distal segment, the *hindgut*, or *endgut*. This differentiation of the tube into successive segments is closely connected with the character and quantity of the food habitually taken and with the method and rapidity of its elaboration in the process of digestion, absorption and excretion. In general the *foregut* is formed by the segment which succeeds to the oral cavity, and includes the *pharynx*, *œsophagus* and *stomach*. The *midgut* is composed of a longer or shorter narrower tube of nearly uniform caliber, the *small intestine*, which follows the gastric dilatation. Even in forms in which the stomach is not distinctly differentiated (cf. p. 40) the connection of the biliary duct with the intestinal canal serves to separate the fore- and midgut. The *hindgut* or *large intestine* is usually separated from the preceding segment by an external circular constriction, with a corresponding annular valve or fold of the mucous membrane in the interior.

The beginning of the large intestine is marked in many forms by the development of an accessory pouch or diverticulum, the *cæcum*. The hindgut extends from its junction with the midgut to the cloacal or anal opening.

1. Midgut or Small Intestine.

The small intestine is the segment of the alimentary canal in which digestion of the non-nitrogenous food substances takes place, and which affords the necessary area of mucous surface for the absorption of all digested matters. Consequently the character and habitual quantity of the food here elaborated exerts a very marked influence on the *length* of the small intestine, *i. e.*, on the extent of the digestive and absorbing surface represented by its mucous membrane.

The relative length of the small intestine in any individual form will vary with both the quantity and volume of the food and with the rapidity of the metabolic processes. Animals, in which digestion is rapid and the usual food small in bulk and concentrated in its nutrient qualities, have a relatively short intestine, while the canal is longer in forms subsisting on food which is bulky and which demands considerable time for its elaboration. Hence we find the relatively shortest intestine in carnivora, the longest in herbivora, while the canal in omnivora occupies an intermediate position in regard to its relative length.

The rapidity of tissue-metabolism also exerts a marked influence on the length and development of this portion of the alimentary canal.

In the warm-blooded animals (mammals and birds) the tissue-changes are constant and rapid and call for a large amount of nutrition within a given period, while the metabolic processes in the cold-blooded vertebrates (reptiles, amphibia and fishes) are slow, these animals being able to go without food for long periods. Consequently in the former class the small intestine is relatively much longer than in the latter. Thus in certain birds and herbivorous mammals the small intestine exceeds the total length of the body many times. This influence of the quantity and quality of the food on the length of the intestinal canal is seen, for example, very well during the course of development in the frog.

The increase in the length of the intestine, and the consequent varying degrees of coiling and convolution, are therefore secondary acquired characters, depending for their development upon the habitual kind and volume of the food. Additional provisions for increasing the efficiency of the digestive apparatus are encountered throughout the whole of the intestinal canal. In many forms the digestive secretory and absorbing area is augmented by the development of folds, valves, diverticula, villi and papillæ from the mucous surface of the intestine. Certain valves and folds, moreover, both control the direction in which the contents of the canal move and retain the same for a longer period in the intestinal segment in which they develop. Such folds appear especially well developed in the intestine of certain cyclostomes, selachians and dipnœans (cf. Figs. 203 and 204). In these forms the alimentary canal is usually short and straight, and the fold which has a typical spiral course and projects far into the lumen of the gut, evidently makes up to a very large extent for the shortness of the intestine, serving the threefold purpose of

(a) Increasing the digestive and absorbing surface;

(b) Prolonging the period of retention of the food-substances in the intestine, and thus increasing the time available for elaboration and absorption.

(c) Regulating the direction in which the intestinal contents move.

We will see presently that a similar spiral mucous fold is also encountered in some of the higher vertebrates, especially in the large intestine. Examples are found in the well-developed spiral valve in the cæca of the ostrich (Fig. 341), the similar fold in the large intestine of many rodents (Figs. 387 and 388) and in the crescentic plicæ of the primate large intestine (Figs. 471, 472 and 473).

To the same physiological category belong the *digestive diverticula* of the intestinal canal, such as the pyloric appendices of the midgut found in many teleosts and ganoids (cf. p. 119) and the varieties of cæca or blind diverticula of the hindgut encountered throughout the vertebrate series. They all function as reservoirs which increase the available digestive and absorbing surface and which in addition are especially adapted to retain substances difficult of digestion until the processes of elaboration have been completed.

Divisions of the Small Intestine.—In the higher forms the segment of the small intestine which succeeds to the pylorus is distinguished as the *duodenum*. Into it empty the ducts of the liver and pancreas. In some animals a pear-shaped enlargement is found, corresponding to the *duodenal antrum* of the human intestine, as the dilated proximal portion of the duodenum immediately beyond the pylorus is called. Examples of this condition are furnished by the cetaceans, several rodents, the llama and dromedary and the koala (Phascolarctos).

In the birds and in many mammals (e. g., dog, Fig. 200, and many rodents, as the rabbit) the duodenum is drawn out into a long loop surrounding the pancreas.

Structure of the Small Intestine. 1. Secretory Apparatus.—The glands whose ducts empty into the small intestine and which furnish the digestive secretions, may be divided as follows:

(a) Glands situated in the substance of the intestinal walls.

Two kinds are distinguished:

1. Brunner's glands, small acinous glands confined to the first part of the duodenum.

2. Glands of Lieberkühn, small cæcal pits distributed not only over the entire small intestine, but also found in the mucous membrane of the large intestine.

These structures furnish the intestinal juice, whose chief function is the conversion of starches into sugar, while aiding in carnivorous animals also the digestion of proteid substances. The glands are hence best developed in herbivora, while in carnivora they are present in diminished numbers since they assist in the digestion of proteid substances.

The size and number of these glands also depends on the amount of food digested within a given period. When a considerable quantity of digestive fluid is required, in order to obtain the nutritive value of the food for the organism rapidly, the glandular apparatus of the intestine will be well developed. Hence mammalia, in whom these conditions exist, possess both the glands of Brunner and of Lieberkühn. In birds the latter structures are still found, but the former are absent, while amphibia and fishes are devoid of both kinds. In these lower vertebrates the typical intestinal glandular apparatus of the higher forms is to a certain

96

extent replaced by small pits and depressions of the mucous membrane bounded by reticular folds.

(b) Glands situated outside the intestinal tube, into whose lumen their ducts empty.

The liver and pancreas fall under this head. The liver functions in the digestion of the fatty substances of the food, while the secretion of the pancreas converts the starches into sugars, and aids in the digestion of albumenoid substances and to a lesser degree in that of the fats.

2. Absorbing Apparatus of Small Intestine.—The mucous membrane of the intestine is provided with villi, containing lymphatics, by whose agency the digested matters are absorbed. These structures are developed in individual forms in direct proportion to the ease and rapidity with which the food is habitually absorbed.

The more rapid and complete the digestion is the greater will be the amount of digested nutritive material at any given time in the intestine, and the greater will be the development of the absorbing structures. Hence the villi of the small intestine are especially large and prominent in the carnivora, while they are small and insignificant in herbivora and omnivora. Intestinal villi are found in nearly all mammals and in many birds. Fig. 300 shows the villi of the intestinal mucous membrane in a carnivore mammal (*Ursus maritimus*, polar bear) and Fig. 301 the same structures in the cassowary (*Casuarius casuarius*) in which bird they are very well developed. The villi are not confined to the two highest vertebrate classes, but are encountered also in the mucous membrane of the midgut in certain reptiles, notably the ophidia.

Fig. 302 shows the intestine mucous membrane of the boa constrictor with well-developed and prominent villous projections.

FIG. 300.—Small intestine, of polar bear, *Ursus maritimus.* Mucous surface. (Columbia University Museum, No. 782.)

FIG. 301.—Duodenum, with entrance of pancreatic and biliary ducts and well-developed diverticulum Vateri in the cassowary, *Casuarius casuarius* (Columbia University Museum, No. 1821.)

FIG. 302.—Mucous membrane of midgut of *Boa constrictor.* (Columbia University Museum, No. 1837.)

FIG. 303.—Mucous surface of small intestine of a species of African antelope, *Cervicapra arundinacea.* (Columbia University Museum, No. 1843.)

FIG. 304.—Mucous surface of small intestine of *Phocæna communis*, porpoise. (Columbia University Museum, No. 1057.)

FIG. 305.—Mucous membrane of mid-gut of *Lophius piscatorius*, the angler, 18 cm. caudad of pylorus. (Columbia University Museum, No. 1838.)

FIGS. 306, 307.—Intestinal mucous membrane of logger-head turtle, *Thalassochelys caretta.* (Columbia University Museum, No. 1839.)

FIG. 306.—Mid-gut.

FIG. 307.—End-gut.

FIG. 308.—Adult human subject. Mucous membrane of pyloro-duodenal junction and of duodenum. (Columbia University Museum, No. 1840.)

FIG. 309.—Adult human subject. Mucous membrane of small intestine, showing arrangement of valvulæ conniventes in successive portions of jejunum and ileum. (Columbia University Museum, No. 1841.)

Some birds, such as the snipes, herons and crows, have in place of the intestinal villi projecting folds of the mucosa, often arranged in a reticular manner. This type is prevalent in amphibia and fish (Fig. 112, distal segment of midgut). Collections of lymphoid tissue in the mucous membrane of the small intestine, either aggregated to form Peyer's patches (Fig. 309) or as solitary follicles, are only found in the two highest vertebrate classes, birds and mammals. In the former they appear scattered over the surface of the mucous membrane, in the latter they may be arranged in aggregations or regular rows. They are not secreting structures, but their exact function in absorption is not known. This lymphoid or adenoid tissue in certain forms is especially well developed at the ileo-colic junction, forming the *lymphatic sac* of some rodents, as lepus (cf. Fig. 386). It is not confined to the small

97

intestine, but is found in the large intestine as well. At times it appears especially well developed in the terminal portion of the cæcal pouch (appendix), as in *Lepus*(Fig. 388).

The *valvulæ conniventes*or *valves of Kerkring* of the human small intestine serve to very greatly increase the secreting and absorbing mucous surface. They are not found in this complete development in any other mammals, although a very few forms present a transverse reduplication of the intestinal mucosa and the circular layer of muscular fibers. An example of this is found in the intestinal mucous membrane of a species of antelope, shown in Fig. 303.

The complete development of the valvulæ conniventes in man is possibly also associated with a mechanical function in connection with the upright posture. In some mammalia, as in certain rodents and the porpoise (Fig. 304), the mucous membrane of the terminal part of the small intestine is thrown into *longitudinal folds*.

The mucosa of the midgut in the lower vertebrates may be smooth, or thrown into longitudinal folds, or the longitudinal folds may become connected by oblique and transverse secondary folds, resulting finally in a more or less complicated reticulated pattern of crypts. A very good example of the type-form from which the more complicated conditions are derived is seen in Fig. 305, showing the mucous membrane of the midgut in*Lophius piscatorius*, the angler. The specimen is taken 18 cm. from the pylorus and shows a ground plan of longitudinal plicæ connected by short oblique cross folds.

Fig. 306, showing the midgut mucosa of the loggerhead turtle (*Thalassochelys caretta*), exhibits the same arrangement further developed, resulting in a fine reticulated pattern, while in the endgut of the same animal the primitive longitudinal folding is resumed (Fig. 307).

The number and size of the human valvulæ conniventes vary in different parts of the small intestine (Fig. 309). They are not usually found in the beginning of the duodenum (Fig. 308), but commence in the second or descending portion.

They become very large and closely packed immediately beyond the common entrance of the biliary and pancreatic ducts and continue to be well developed and numerous throughout the rest of the duodenum and upper half of the jejunum (Figs. 308 and 309). From here on they become smaller, more irregular and less closely packed, and finally in the terminal two feet of the ileum disappear almost entirely (Fig. 309). This varying development of the valvulæ is the chief reason why a given segment of the ileum weighs less than a corresponding length of the jejunum. This reduction in the fold-formation of the intestinal mucosa toward the terminal portion of the midgut is seen even in the lower vertebrates. Thus in Fig. 112, showing the entire intestinal tract of the conger eel, *Echelus conger*, in section, the plicæ of the mucous membrane in the proximal segment of the midgut, at and immediately beyond the entrance of the biliary duct, are prominent and numerous. This redundancy continues but slightly reduced in the descending limb of the intestinal loop, while in the ascending limb and up to the ileo-colic junction the folds are reduced to a fine reticulated meshwork. Beyond the ileo-colic valve plate, in the short endgut, the mucosa again presents numerous pointed reduplications.

II. ENDGUT OR LARGE INTESTINE.

In this segment of the intestinal canal the undigested remnants of the food are collected and evacuated from time to time.

In addition, the mucous membrane of the large intestine absorbs all *digested* material which is passed from the small intestine. While digestion of food-substances will not be*inaugurated* in the large intestine, material already in the process of digestion and mixed with the intestinal juices of the preceding segment, will be further elaborated in this portion of the canal and the nutritive products absorbed. This is especially the case in herbivora and omnivora, whose food is bulky, containing a large amount of refuse material, and is hence only slowly digested. On the other hand the food of the carnivora is easily and rapidly digested and absorbed. After passing through the small intestine hardly any substances remain which are capable of digestion and absorption. Hence the large intestine of herbivora and omnivora is uniformly longer in proportion to the small intestine than it is in carnivorous animals. In the former this segment of the canal functions as an accessory digestive apparatus and hence, as we will see, often develops accessory structural modifications, such as a large cæcum and spiral colon, while in the latter it acts almost solely as a canal for the evacuation of the indigestible remnants.

Again, the large intestine is better developed in the higher animals, in mammalia and to a lesser degree in birds, in whom the functional demands for nutrition are active and require that a relatively large amount of food should pass through the digestive tract in a given time. On the other hand in the lower cold-blooded vertebrates the metabolism is less active, less food is taken and it is not necessary to secure all the nutrient material contained in the same for the organism. The great differences observed in the vertebrate series in regard to length, width and structure of the large intestine depend upon these physiological conditions. The divisions of the human large intestine into cæcum, ascending, transverse and descending colon, sigmoid flexure and rectum are found only in the primates, and here not uniformly.

In the lower vertebrate classes the endgut is very short, corresponding only to the pelvic segment of the Mammalia (rectum), a colon proper being absent in these forms (cf. Fig. 112,*Echelus conger*). The human large intestine exhibits a very characteristic structure. Throughout the greater part of the colon the longitudinal muscular layer is mainly disposed in the form of three bands or tænia (ligamenta coli). The canal itself is longer than these bands, thus producing a folding of the walls in the form of three rows of pouches (cellulæ coli), in the intervals between the bands. The pouches of each row are separated from each other externally by constrictions, internally by projecting crescentic folds (plicæ coli) (Figs. 471, 472 and 474).

This arrangement of the large intestine is also found in the monkeys (Fig. 473) and in certain Rodents (Fig. 474).

In other mammals the large intestine is smooth and cylindrical and the longitudinal layer of muscular fibers uniform (Fig. 475).

In general the vertebrate large intestine is *wider* than the small, usually in the proportion of 5:1 or 6:1.

In some ruminant Herbivora, however, the great length of the colon leads to a reduction of the caliber in certain segments so that the large intestine does not exceed the width of the small, or even falls below the same.

The *length* of the large intestine, as in man, is usually much less than that of the small intestine. As already stated this disproportion is more marked in Carnivora than in Herbivora.

The ratio in length of the large to the small intestine is very low in the Seals (1:14), and in several Edentates, as *Myrmecophaga*, *Tamandua* and *Bradypus* (1:9-11).

In the carnivorous mammals it ranges 1:5-7.

In some of the ruminant Herbivora, as the cow and sheep, it is 1:4, while in the deer, horse, certain Rodents (as *Lepus* and *Cricetus*) it reaches as high as 1:2 or 1:3.

The large intestine is usually relatively short in birds, reptiles, amphibia and fish.

In the Cassowary the length of the large to the small intestine is 1:6.

In some of the birds of prey (eagle) the proportion falls as low as 1:68 or 70.

Exceptions to the general rule are furnished by some of the herbivorous Cetaceans and by the Dugong (*Halicore*) in whom the large intestine is twice as long as the small. Again in the Ostrich the large intestine in one example measured 40', while the length of the small intestine was only 22'. This unusual development of the large intestine indicates the necessity of retaining the food, which is bulky and difficult of digestion, until the elaboration is completed. The same significance belongs to the enormously developed cæca of these birds (cf. p. 204).

The separation of the small and large intestine is marked externally by the *cæcum*, when present, and internally by the *valve of the colon*. The details of the vertebrate ileo-colic junction will be considered in the following pages.

II. SERIAL REVIEW OF THE ILEO-COLIC JUNCTION AND CONNECTED
STRUCTURES IN VERTEBRATES.
I. FISHES.

In the Cyclostomata there is no differentiation between the mid- and hindgut. Fig. 310shows the entire alimentary canal of *Petromyzon marinus*, the lamprey, caudad of the pericardium.

In some fishes the midgut is differentiated from the hindgut by an external circular constriction, corresponding to an annular projecting fold of the mucosa in the interior which resembles the pyloro-duodenal valve. There is no cæcum, and the short hindgut empties into the cephalic and ventral aspect of the cloaca. Fig. 311 shows the entire intestinal tract of a Teleost fish, *Echelus conger*, the conger eel. The midgut, provided at the beginning with a short globular pyloric appendix (cf. p. 119), constitutes the longest individual segment of the canal. The hindgut, separated from the preceding by a constriction, is very short and of large caliber. Fig. 312 shows the broad annular valve with central circular opening which separates mid- and hindgut in the interior, and Fig. 313 the ileo-colic junction in section in the same animal.

FIG. 310.—*Petromyzon marinus*, lamprey. Entire alimentary canal below pericardium. (Columbia University Museum, No. 1575.)

FIG. 311.—*Echelus conger*, Conger eel. Alimentary canal, stomach, mid- and hindgut, liver, and spleen. (Columbia University Museum, No. 1430.)

FIG. 312.—*Echelus conger*, Conger eel. Ileo-colic junction, opened. (Columbia University Museum, No. 1434.)

FIG. 313.—*Echelus conger*, Conger eel. Section of mid- and end-gut, with ileo-colic junction, hardened. (Columbia University Museum, No. 1349.)

FIG. 314.—*Gadus callarias*, cod-fish. Ileo-colic junction. Intestine on each side opened, with probe passed through constricted opening of ileo-colic valve. (Columbia University Museum, No. 1260.)

FIG. 315.—*Pleuronectes maculatus*, flounder. Ileo-colon, opened to show ileo-colic valve. (Columbia University Museum, No. 1493.)

FIG. 316.—*Galeus canis*, dog-shark, ♂. Genito-urinary tract and cloaca *in situ*. (Columbia University Museum, No. 1694.)

FIG. 317.—*Accipenser sturio*, sturgeon. Alimentary canal. (Columbia University Museum, Nos. 1826, 1827, and 1828.)

A similar type of ileo-colic junction is seen in other Teleosts, as in *Gadus callarias*, the cod (Fig. 314), *Pleuronectes maculatus*, the flounder (Fig. 315), and in some Ganoids, as *Accipenser sturio*, the sturgeon (Fig. 212). In some Selachians an appendicular diverticulum, the so-called "rectal" or "digitiform gland," is found connected with the terminal segment of the gut near the entrance of the same into the cloaca (Fig. 316).

II. AMPHIBIA.

The alimentary canal is simple and usually comparatively short. There is no cæcal pouch. Differentiation of mid- and endgut is usually marked externally by a constriction and by the increased caliber of the terminal intestinal segment.

FIG. 318.—*Rana catesbiana*, bull-frog. Alimentary canal and appendages. (Columbia University Museum, No. 1454.)

FIG. 319.—*Necturus maculatus*, mud-puppy. Alimentary canal and appendages. (Columbia University Museum, No. 1582.)

FIG. 320.—*Cryptobranchus alleghaniensis*, hellbender. Ileo-colic junction. (Columbia University Museum, No. 1711.)

Fig. 318 shows the alimentary canal of the bull-frog, *Rana catesbiana*, Fig. 319 that of a Urodele Amphibian, *Necturus maculatus*, and Fig. 320 the ileo-colic junction isolated in *Cryptobranchus alleghaniensis*, the hellbender.

III. REPTILIA.

In reptiles a well-marked differentiation of small and large intestine is the rule.

Four types of ileo-colic junction are encountered in this class:

1. The transition from small to large intestine is marked by the greatly increased caliber of the latter and by an annular valve in the interior. An example of this type is furnished by *Alligator mississippiensis* (Fig. 321) and a similar form is encountered in some lizards, as *Heloderma suspectum*, the Gila monster (Fig. 322).

FIG. 321.—*Alligator mississippiensis,* alligator. Ileo-colon; dried preparation. (Columbia University Museum, No. 179.)

FIG. 322.—*Heloderma suspectum,* Gila monster. (Columbia University Museum, No. 69/1536.)

2. The large intestine immediately beyond the ileo-colic junction protrudes along the convex border to form a rudimentary lateral cæcum. This type is found in many Chelonians, *e. g.*, in *Pseudemys elegans*, the pond turtle (Figs. 323 and 324) and *Chelydra serpentaria*, the snapping turtle (Fig. 325).

FIG. 323.—*Pseudemys elegans,* pond-turtle. (Columbia University Museum, No. 1069.)

FIG. 324.—*Pseudemys elegans,* pond-turtle. Ileo-colic junction, opened. (Columbia University Museum, No. 1524.)

FIG. 325.—*Chelydra serpentaria*, snapping turtle. Intestinal canal, pancreas, and spleen. (Columbia University Museum, No. 1369.)

FIG. 326.—*Iguana tuberculata*, iguana. Ileo-colic junction and cæcum; dried preparation. (Columbia University Museum, No. 243.)

3. The ileo-colic junction is provided with a well-developed sacculated cæcal pouch derived from the proximal segment of the colon and divided in the interior by folds into several secondary compartments.

This type is found in some of the phytophagous lizards, as *Iguana tuberculata* (Figs. 326 and 327). The small intestine of this animal is of considerable length and of uniform caliber from the pylorus to the ileo-colic junction. The cæcum is a large sacculated pouch developed chiefly along the convex border of the large intestine opposite to the mesenteric attachment.

FIG. 327.—*Iguana tuberculata*, iguana. Mid-gut, ileo-colic junction, cæcum, and end-gut; dried preparation. (Columbia University Museum, No. 178.)

FIG. 329.—Drawing taken from same preparation (No. 1321) to elucidate more clearly internal structure of cæcal pouch.

FIG. 328.—*Iguana tuberculata*, iguana. Ileo-colic junction and cæcum in section. (Columbia University Museum, No. 1321.)

FIG. 330.—*Cyclura teres*, smooth-backed cyclura. Ileo-colic junction and cæcum in section. (Columbia University Museum, No. 1523.)

The examination of the interior of this pouch reveals a complicated structure (Figs. 328 and 329). Fig. 330 shows the same structures in a closely allied form, *Cyclura teres*. The entrance of the small intestine is guarded by an annular sphincter valve, whose central circular opening leads into a proximal compartment of the cæcum. This compartment is in turn separated from the remainder of the cæcal pouch by a second circular valvular fold with central opening. Beyond this valve the interior of the pouch carries a number of crescentic mucous folds, corresponding to the external constrictions between the cæcal sacculations. The entire pouch gradually diminishes in caliber and finally passes with a sharp angular bend into the terminal portion of the endgut. At this point the lumen of the canal is slightly diminished by a sphincter-like thickening of the muscularis, producing an annular projection of the mucous membrane. The entire cæcal pouch appears as a specialized segment of the large intestine interposed between the termination of the midgut and the terminal portion of the endgut, which latter is characterized by uniform caliber and increased thickness of the muscular walls.

The highly developed and complicated structure of the cæcal apparatus in *Iguana* and allied forms exemplifies very clearly the influence of *vegetable* food on the development of this segment of the alimentary tract when compared with the simple type of ileo-colic transition found in *carnivorous* lizards, as *Heloderma* (Fig. 322). *Iguana* subsists on leaves, fruits and other vegetable matter and the cæcal pouch is invariably found filled with the firmer and less digestible portions of this food. These are undoubtedly retained in the pouch by the series of valves and folds until digestion and absorption of all available nutritive material forwarded from the small intestine is completed. On the other hand *Heloderma* lives almost entirely on bird eggs, a concentrated and easily digested food. Consequently the ileo-colic junction in this lizard is exceedingly simple and rudimentary, marked merely by a slight external constriction, with an annular valve in the interior, and an increase in the caliber of the short hindgut, resembling the form found in many teleost fishes.

4. Finally in some Ophidians a typical lateral cæcal pouch of considerable dimensions is found connected with the endgut immediately beyond the ileo-colic junction.

An example of this reptilian type, closely resembling the corresponding structure in many Mammalia, is presented by *Eunectes marinus*, the anaconda, shown in Figs. 331 and 332.

FIG. 331.—*Eunectes marinus*, anaconda. Mid- and end-gut, with ileo-colic junction and cæcum. (Columbia University Museum, No. 72/1535.)

FIG. 332.—*Eunectes marinus*, anaconda. Mid- and end-gut, with ileo-colic junction and cæcum laid open. (Columbia University Museum, No. 1709.)

IV. ILEO-COLIC JUNCTION IN BIRDS.

In the birds the length of the intestine is subject to great variations. The canal is short in species subsisting on fruits and insects, long in those feeding on seeds, plants and fish. The large intestine, immediately beyond the ileo-colic junction, is provided typically with two symmetrical lateral cæca which extend in some forms for a considerable distance cephalad on each side of the small intestine to which they are bound by peritoneal connections.

FIG. 333.—*Buteo harloni*, black hawk. Ileo-colic junction and cæca. (Columbia University Museum, No. 1502.)

FIG. 334.—*Phalacrocorax dilophus*, double-crested cormorant. Ileo-colic junction and cæca. (Columbia University Museum, No. 67/1534.)

As a rule carnivorous birds have short and rudimentary pouches (Figs. 333 and 334), whereas they are long in herbivorous forms (Figs. 335 and 336). Some carnivorous birds, as*Corvus, Strix*, etc., have fairly long cæca (Fig. 337). In the passerine birds living on seeds and insects, the cæca are of considerable length as they are also in some of the piscivorous divers (Figs. 338 and 339). They are long in the Ratitæ, and in the Lamellirostra, who feed chiefly on plants (Fig. 340).

FIG. 335.—*Gallus bankiva*, hen. Ileo-colic junction and cæca. (Columbia University Museum, No. 1486.)

FIG. 337.—*Bubo virginianus*, great horned owl. Ileo-colic junction and cæca. (Columbia University Museum, No. 672.)

FIG. 336.—*Chen hyperborea*, Canada snow-goose, Ileo-colic junction and cæca. (Columbia University Museum, No. 47/1448.)

FIG. 338.—*Urinator lumme*, red-throated loon. Ileo-colic junction and cæca. (Columbia University Museum, No. 1001.)

FIG. 339.—*Merganser serrator*, red-breasted merganser. Ileo-colic junction and cæca. (Columbia

FIG. 340.—*Casuarius casuarius*, cassowary. (Columbia University

102

University Museum, No. 1798.)

Museum, No. 1799.)

FIG. 341.—*Struthio africanus*, African ostrich. Ileo-colic junction and cæca. (Columbia University Museum, No. 48/1573.)

FIG. 342.—*Ardea virescens*, green heron. Ileo-colic junction and cæcum. (Columbia University Museum, No. 1132 a.)

The enormously elongated cæca of the African ostrich contain a spiral fold of the mucous membrane in the interior (Fig. 341).

In place of the usual double avian cæcum a single pouch is found in a few forms, namely in the Herons (Fig. 342).

FIG. 344.—*Urinator imber*, great northern diver. Small intestine with cæcal pouch; the remnant of the vitello-intestinal duct. (Columbia University Museum, No. 78/1573)

FIG. 343.—*Urinator lumme*, red-throated loon. Small intestine with cæcal pouch; the remnant of the vitello-intestinal duct. (Columbia University Museum, No. 997.)

In some birds the small intestine is also provided with a cæcal pouch, the remnant of the vitello-intestinal duct corresponding in its significance to the occasional mammalian diverticulum of Meckel (Figs. 343 and 344). (cf. p. 35.)

V. ILEO-COLIC JUNCTION, CÆCUM AND VERMIFORM APPENDIX IN THE MAMMALIA.

I. Subclass: Ornithodelphia.
I. Order: Monotremata.

In many particulars the anatomical structure of these animals reveals a close relationship to the Sauropsida. They represent the mammalian class in its lowest stage of evolution.

The ileo-colic junction in all the existing forms is direct, without angular bend at the entrance of the small into the large intestine. The cæcum is a long narrow pouch, slightly dilated at the extremity, derived from the beginning of the colon and extending backward along the free margin of the small intestine. The cæcum resembles in its general shape and structure the pouches seen in many birds, except that it is unilateral, while the birds normally have two symmetrical cæca. The cæcum of *Ornithorhynchus anatinus*, the platypus or duck bill, is shown in Figs. 345 and 346, and that of *Echidna hystrix*, the spiny ant-eater, in Fig. 347. These two animals represent the two genera into which the order is divided.

FIG. 345.—*Ornithorhynchus anatinus*, duck mole. Ileo-colon and cæcum. (Columbia University Museum, No. 1499.)

FIG. 346.—*Ornithorhynchus anatinus*, duck mole. Ileo-colon and cæcum. (Columbia University Museum, No. 1500.)

FIG. 347.—*Echidna hystrix*, spiny ant-eater. Ileo-colon and cæcum. (Columbia University Museum, No. 1501.)

II. Subclass: Didelphia.
II. Order: Marsupialia.

FIG. 348.—*Didelphis virginiana*, opossum. Ileo-colic junction and cæcum. (Columbia University Museum, No. 1533.)

The Didelphia are represented by numerous species, which are united by certain common anatomical characters of the reproductive organs and dentition to form the order of the Marsupialia. The individual species included within this order differ widely in abit, food, mode of locomotion, etc., and consequently exhibit great diversity in the structure of the skeletal and muscular systems and of the alimentary canal. With the exception of the Opossums inhabiting the new world, the families composing the order are confined to the Australian continent and the adjacent islands. In respect to the alimentary tract in general and the ileo-colic junction in particular, we are evidently dealing with a group of animals which, while they retain the common characters above indicated as uniting them in the marsupial order, yet have in the structure of their digestive canal adapted themselves to widely divergent conditions of food supply and environment. Consequently within the confines of this single and largely isolated order, we encounter nearly all the types of cæcum and ileo-colic junction which are found among the remaining mammalia. The group in its individual representatives has passed, so to speak, through the different stages of development and evolution which, on a very much larger scale, are exhibited by the remaining mammalian orders.

We can, independently of the systematic zoölogical classification, arrange the forms composing the order under the following types:

1. *Forms with large well-developed simple cæca, of uniform caliber, with rounded globular termination.*

This type is encountered among the herbivorous Marsupials, such as the opossums, kangaroos and wallabys. Fig. 348 shows the structures in *Didelphis virginiana*, the common opossum, Fig. 349 in a small species of opossum from Trinidad, and Fig. 350 the same parts in *Halmaturus derbyanus*, the rock wallaby.

FIG. 349.—*Didelphis sp.?* opossum. Ileo-colic junction and cæcum. (Columbia University, Study Collection.)

FIG. 350.—*Halmaturus derbyanus*, rock kangaroo. Ileo-colic junction and cæcum. (Columbia University Museum, No. 727.)

2. *Forms with enormously developed sacculated cæca, coiled spirally, with or without additional convolutions of the proximal colon; the terminal portion of the cæcal pouch diminishes in caliber to form a pointed appendage.*

This type of cæcum characterizes the *Phalangeridæ* or Phalangers and the *Phascolarctidæ*.

Examples are shown in Figs. 351 and 352, representing the structures in *Trichosurus vulpinus*, the vulpine phalanger, and *Phascolarctos cinereus*, the koala.

FIG. 351.—*Trichosurus vulpinus*, vulpine phalanger. Ileo-colic junction and cæcum. (Columbia University Museum, No. 1800.)

FIG. 352.—*Phascolarctos cinereus*, koala. Ileo-colic junction and cæcum. (Drawn from preparation.) (Columbia University Museum, No. 1528.)

3. *Forms with simple cæca of moderate size.*

The *Peramelidæ* or bandicoots.

Fig. 353 shows the ileo-colic junction, cæcum and proximal segment of the colon in *Perameles nasuta*, the bandicoot.

FIG. 353.—*Perameles nasuta*, bandicoot. Ileo-colic junction and cæcum. (Columbia University Museum, No. 1481.)

4. *Forms with sacculated short cæca, whose terminal portion is reduced to constitute a typical vermiform appendix.*

The cæcum of the *Phascolomyidæ* or wombats, resembles, in its general structure and in the presence of a typical vermiform appendix, very closely the corresponding parts of the alimentary canal in man and the anthropoid apes. Fig. 354 shows these structures in *Phascolomys wombat*, the common wombat.

FIG. 354.—*Phascolomys wombat*, wombat. Ileo-cæcum and appendix. (Columbia University Museum, No. 1508.)

5. *Forms with simple direct ileo-colic junction without cæcum.*

In the purely carnivorous Marsupials, comprising the family of the *Dasyuridæ*, the reduction of the cæcal apparatus, foreshadowed by the appearance of the distal rudimentary segment as a vermiform appendix in the wombats, has been carried to the complete elimination of the pouch. The ileo-colic junction in these animals is simple, marked externally by a circular constriction and internally by an annular valve. The colon forms a very short terminal segment of the alimentary canal. The parts are shown in Fig. 355 in a typical representative of the family, *Dasyurus viverinus*, the Tasmanian devil.

FIG. 355.—*Dasyurus viverinus*, dasyurus, Tasmanian devil. Intestinal canal. Ileo-colic junction. (Columbia University Museum, No. 1463.)

The structural modifications encountered in the digestive tract of these carnivorous Marsupials can properly be regarded as the result of their habitual diet, and we will meet with analogous and identical examples of cæcal reduction in the typical Carnivores among the placental mammals (cf. p. 212).

III. Subclass: Monodelphia.
III. Order: Edentata.

In all probability the Sloths, Ant-eaters and Armadillos composing this order represent a highly specialized remnant of an ancient group now largely extinct. In respect to the ileo-colic junction the Edentates may be arranged in two groups which offer, within the limited number of existing species, a very complete transitional series.

I. SYMMETRICAL TYPE OF ILEO-COLIC JUNCTION.

1. *Differentiation in caliber, with direct funnel-like transition of small into large intestine. No cæcum.*

Beyond the ileo-colic junction the caliber of the large intestine increases gradually. The terminal ileum is thus implanted into the apex of a funnel formed by the proximal segment of the colon.

Examples of this type are furnished by *Myrmecophaga jubata*, the great ant-eater (Fig. 356), and by *Cholæpus didactylus*, the two-toed sloth (Fig. 357).

FIG. 356.—*Myrmecophaga jubata*, great ant-eater. Ileo-colic junction. (Columbia University Museum, No. 1519.)

FIG. 357.—*Cholæpus didactylus*, two-toed sloth. Ileo-colic junction. (Columbia University Museum, No. 714.)

FIG. 358.—*Tatusia novemcincta*, nine-banded armadillo. Ileo-colic junction. (Columbia University Museum, No. 176.)

2. *Abrupt demarcation of small and large intestine, with median transition of ileum.*

The caliber of the intestine enlarges rapidly immediately beyond the ileo-colic junction. This form is derived from the preceding by the substitution of the abrupt ileo-colic transition for the gradual funnel-shaped development of the large intestine.

The type is illustrated by *Tatusia novemcincta*, the nine-banded armadillo (Fig. 358), and is also found in two other armadillos, *Tolypeutes* and *Xenurus*.

3. *The colon on each side of the ileo-colic junction is prolonged backward along the small intestine, forming two symmetrical lateral globular colic cæca.*

This type, which is to be regarded as a further development of the preceding form, is also found in the armadillos. Fig. 359 represents the structures in *Dasypus sexcinctus*, the six-banded armadillo, and a similar arrangement of the parts exists in *Chlamydophorus*, another species of armadillo.

FIG. 359.—*Dasypus sexcinctus*, six-banded armadillo, Ileo-colic junction and cæca. (Columbia University Museum, No. 1478.)

4. *The cæcal pouches are more completely differentiated, communicating with the colon by a constricted neck.*

This results in an arrangement which recalls the structure of many avian cæca (cf. Fig. 337) and is seen in the double cæcal pouches of *Cyclothurus didactylus*, the little ant-eater (Fig. 360).

FIG. 360.—*Cyclothurus didactylus*, little ant-eater. Ileo-colic junction and cæca. (Columbia University Museum, No. 1512.)

II. ASYMMETRICAL TYPE OF ILEO-COLIC JUNCTION.

The second general group of the Edentates is characterized by the gradual development of a single lateral asymmetrical cæcum, in place of the median symmetrical ileo-colic transition found in the forms just considered. The species composing this group thus form a link leading up to the right-angled accession of ileum to large intestine and the lateral cæcum characteristic of most other mammalia.

FIG. 361.—*Manis longicauda*, long-tailed pangolin. Ileo-colic junction; dry preparation. (Columbia University Museum, No. 95.)

FIG. 362.—*Manis longicauda*, long-tailed pangolin. Ileo-colic junction. (Columbia University Museum, No. 328.)

FIG. 363.—*Arctopithecus marmoratus*, three-toed sloth. Ileo-colic junction. (Columbia University Museum, No. 1479.)

1. This type may be considered as being inaugurated by the form of ileo-colic junction found in the *Manidæ* or *Pangolins*, as illustrated by Figs. 361 and 362, taken from the long-tailed pangolin, *Manis longicauda.* There is no cæcum and only a slight differentiation in caliber between the small and large intestine. The gut in all the forms examined shows a very characteristic bend at the ileo-colic junction, being twisted into a figure of 8 and held in place by mesenteric folds.

2. The second stage, illustrated by *Arctopithecus (Bradypus) marmoratus*, the three-toed sloth (Fig. 363), reveals a distinct increase in the caliber and convexity of the large intestine opposite the mesenteric border immediately beyond the ileo-colic junction.

3. This leads in the third stage, represented by *Tamandua bivittata*, the Tamandua ant-eater (Figs. 364 and 365), to the development of a distinct lateral cæcal pouch. I have had no opportunity of examining the structures in *Orycteropus*, but from the published descriptions[8] the large cæcum of this animal would form the final link in this series.

FIG. 364.—*Tamandua bivittata*, Tamandua ant-eater. Ileo-colic junction and cæcum. (Columbia University Museum, No. 1590.)

FIG. 365.—*Tamandua bivittata*, Tamandua ant-eater. Ventral view of abdominal viscera from the left side. (Study Collection, Columbia University.)

IV. Order: Sirenia.

Of the two living representatives of this remarkable mammalian order the dugong (*Halicore*) is described as possessing a single cæcum, while the cæcal pouch of *Manatus americanus*, the manatee, is symmetrically bifid at the extremity (Fig. 366).

FIG. 366.—*Manatus americanus*, American manatee. Ileo-colic junction and bifid cæcum. (Columbia University Museum, No. 673.)

V. Order: Cetacea.

In the majority of the whales the ileo-colic junction is simple without cæcum, as in *Physeter, Delphinus, Monodon* and *Phocæna* (Fig. 367).

FIG. 367.—*Phocæna communis*, porpoise. Ileo-colic junction. (Columbia University Museum, No. 1007.)

A few forms have a small cæcal pouch.

VI. Order: Ungulata.

The intestinal canal, in conformity with the herbivorous habit of the group, is uniformly provided with a large cæcum, and in many forms the proximal segment of the colon immediately beyond the ileo-colic junction is more or less extensively coiled in a spiral manner. This arrangement is, without doubt, to be regarded as being functionally accessory to the cæcal apparatus, in the sense of increasing very much the area of the secreting and absorbing surface and of prolonging the period during which food-substances, which are slow and difficult of elaboration, are retained in this segment of the alimentary canal.

1. SUBORDER: ARTIODACTYLA.

A. NON-RUMINANTIA.—In the *Suidæ* the cæcum is large and the spiral colon well developed (Fig. 368).

FIG. 368.—*Sus scrofa fœt*, fœtal pig. Ileo-cæcum and spiral colon *in situ*. (Columbia University Museum, No. 1111.)

In the peccaries (*Dicotyles*) the terminal portion of the cæcal pouch is reduced, constituting a centrally implanted appendage.

FIG. 369.—*Dicotyles torquatus*, collared peccary. Ileo-colic junction, cæcum, and spiral colon. (Columbia University Museum, No. 60/1462)

Fig. 369 shows the ileo-colic junction and spiral colon in *Dicotyles torquatus*, the collared peccary, and Fig. 370 the cæcum and appendix of the same animal detached from the spiral colon. In the hippopotamus, on the other hand, the cæcum is said to be absent. If this is the case the animal forms an isolated exception among the Ungulates.

FIG. 370.—*Dicotyles torquatus*, collared peccary. Ileo-colic junction and cæcum, isolated. (Columbia University Museum, No. 1464.)

B. RUMINANTIA.—The cæcum is very large and the spiral coil of the colon extensive.

FIG. 371.—*Capra ægagrus*, Bezoar goat. Ileo-colic junction and cæcum, isolated; dried preparation. (Columbia University Museum, No. 194.)

Fig. 371 shows the cæcum of *Capra ægagrus*, the Bezoar goat, detached from the adjacent intestine, and illustrates the type of the ruminant pouch, of considerable length and caliber, without terminal reduction. The same parts in a preparation of *Boselaphus tragocamelus*, the nilghai, are shown in Fig. 372.

FIG. 372.—*Boselaphus tragocamelus*, nilghai. Ileo-colic junction and cæcum, isolated. (Columbia University, Study Collection.)

FIG. 373.—*Bos indicus*, zebu. Ileo-colic junction, cæcum, and spiral colon. (Columbia University Museum, No. 676.)

Fig. 373 shows the cæcum and ileo-colic junction, together with the spiral coil of the colon, in *Bos indicus*, the zebu, and Fig. 374 the same structures with a typical example of the spiral colon from *Cervus sika*, the Japanese deer; Fig. 375 is taken from a preparation of the parts in a fœtal sheep, while Fig. 376 shows the spiral colon isolated in *Oryx leucoryx*, the oryx.

FIG. 374.—*Cervus sika*, Japanese deer. Ileo-colic junction, cæcum, and spiral colon. (Columbia University, Study Collection.)

FIG. 375.—*Oris aries fœt*, fœtal sheep. Ileo-colic junction, cæcum, and spiral colon. (Columbia University Museum, No. 1379.)

FIG. 376.—*Oryx leucoryx*, oryx. Spiral colon, isolated. (Columbia University, Study Collection.)

2. SUBORDER: PERISSODACTYLA.

In the horse and the rhinoceros the cæcum is very large and of uniform caliber.

FIG. 377.—*Tapirus americanus*, American tapir. Ileo-colic junction, cæcum, and colon. (Columbia University Museum, No. 624.)

In the American tapir (Fig. 377) the large cæcum tapers at its extremity, to form a species of rudimentary appendix, resembling somewhat the corresponding structure in *Dicotyles* (cf.Figs. 369 and 370). The proximal segment of the colon is bent on itself in the form of an extensive loop with closely adherent limbs, illustrating an early stage in the development of the ruminant spiral colon (cf. p. 233).

3. SUBORDER: HYRACOIDEA.

FIG. 378.—*Hyrax syriacus*, hyrax or coney. Intestinal canal, with ileo-colic junction, proximal ileo-colic cæcum, and distal paired colic cæca. (Columbia University, Study Collection.)

FIG. 379.—*Elephas indicus*, Asiatic elephant. Ileo-colic junction and cæcum. (Columbia University Museum, No. 995.)

FIG. 380.—*Myoxus avellanarius*, common dormouse. Alimentary canal. (Columbia University Museum, No. 1466.)

This suborder is formed by the single family of the *Hyracidæ*. In addition to their other isolated and puzzling structural peculiarities the members of this small group present a most unusual arrangement of the intestinal canal, which is unique among living mammalia. In addition to a large sacculated cæcal pouch, situated in the usual position at the beginning of the colon, the large intestine is provided further on with two supplementary elongated pointed conical pouches (Fig. 378).

This unique arrangement, which is not found in any other known vertebrate, may possibly be led back to a type-form encountered in certain saurians (see p. 234).

4. SUBORDER: PROBOSCIDEA.

The cæcum of the elephant is a very large sacculated pouch with rounded termination, illustrated in Fig. 379, taken from the Asiatic elephant.

VII. Order: Rodentia.

With the exception of a single group, the dormice (*Myoxus*) (Fig. 380), the rodents possess a well-developed cæcal apparatus.

In some forms the terminal portion of the pouch is reduced so as to constitute an appendix. Many of these animals, in addition to the cæcum proper, have the proximal colon elongated and coiled in a spiral, and in some this part of the large intestine is provided in the interior with a spiral mucous fold. This latter structure functions again to increase the extent

107

of the mucous absorbing surface and to prolong the retention of substances undergoing slow digestion and absorption.

Typical examples of the capacious sacculated rodent cæcum, with a terminal pointed reduced segment, are afforded by *Castor fiber*, the beaver (Figs. 381 and 382) and by*Erethizon dorsatus*, the Canadian porcupine (Figs. 383 and 384). Figs. 385 and 386 show the ileo-colic junction, cæcum and appendix in *Lepus cuniculus*, the rabbit. The interior of the cæcal pouch and of the proximal segment of the colon is provided with a complete spiral valve (Fig. 387), while the appendix is differentiated by the histological character of its mucous membrane which is studded with closely packed adenoid follicles (Fig. 388). A similar aggregation of lymphoid tissue is found in this animal at the ileo-colic junction forming the s. c. *saccus lymphaticus* (Fig. 387).

FIG. 381.—*Castor fiber*, beaver. Ileo-colic junction, cæcum, and proximal colon; ventral view. (Columbia University Museum, No. 1607.)

FIG. 382.—*Castor fiber*, beaver. Ileo-colic junction, cæcum, and proximal colon; dorsal view. (Columbia University Museum, No. 1607.)

FIG. 383.—*Erethizon dorsatus*, Canadian porcupine. Ileo-colic junction, cæcum, and colon; ventral view. (Columbia University, Study Collection.)

FIG. 384.—*Erethizon dorsatus*, Canadian porcupine. Ileo-colic junction, cæcum, and colon; dorsal view. (Columbia University, Study Collection.)

FIG. 385.—*Lepus cuniculus*, rabbit. Ileo-colic junction and cæcum. (Columbia University Museum, No. 1568.)

FIG. 386.—*Lepus cuniculus*, rabbit. Ileo-colic junction with saccus lymphaticus, isolated, (Columbia University, Study Collection.)

FIG. 387.—*Lepus cuniculus*, rabbit. Ileo-colic junction with saccus lymphaticus. Cæcum and proximal segment of colon opened to show spiral mucous fold in interior. (Columbia University Museum, No. 1587.)

FIG. 388.—*Lepus cuniculus*, rabbit. Cæcum and appendix inverted to show spiral fold and structure of mucosa. (Columbia University Museum, No. 1588.)

The coils of the proximal colon encountered in many rodents are well seen in *Dasyprocta agouti*, the agouti (Figs. 389 and 390), which animal also illustrates a type of cæcum found in several members of the order. The pouch here is large, sacculated, uncinate, without reduction of the terminal portion.

FIG. 389.—*Dasyprocta agouti*, agouti. Ileo-colic junction, cæcum, and colon. (Columbia University Museum, No. 24/1576.)

FIG. 390.—*Dasyprocta agouti*, agouti. Ileo-colic junction, cæcum, and colon. (Drawing based on preparation shown in Fig. 388.)

FIG. 391.—*Lagomys pusillus*. Ileo-colic junction, cæcum, and colon. (After Pallas, from Oppel, "Lehrbuch d. Vergl. mikrosk. Anat. d. Wirbelthiere," II., Jena, 1897, p. 577, Fig. 314.)

FIG. 392.—*Arvicola pennsylvanicus*, field mouse. Alimentary canal. (Columbia University Museum, No. 815.)

FIG. 393.—*Mus decumanus*, white rat. Ileo-colic junction, cæcum, and colon. (Columbia University Museum, No. 1574.)

The relatively enormous size of the cæcum in the *Muridæ* is shown in Fig. 392, representing the entire visceral tract of *Arvicola pennsylvanicus*, the meadow mouse. The pouch in these animals is large, smooth and of uniform caliber (Fig. 393).

In some the colon beyond the entrance of the small intestine is provided with a spiral mucous valve (Fig. 394).

FIG. 394.—*Arvicola riparius*, meadow mouse. Ileo-colic junction, cæcum, and colon. (Columbia University, Study Collection.)

In the single instance of *Myoxus* among the rodents, the ileo-colic junction is simple, without any cæcal pouch (Fig. 380).

VIII. Order: Carnivora.

A. PINNIPEDIA.—In the seals and walrus the cæcum is very small with a blunt termination. Fig. 395 shows its structure in *Zalophus gillespiei*, Gillespie's sea-lion, and Fig. 396 in*Phoca vitulina*, the harbor seal.

108

FIG. 395.—*Zalophus gillespiei*, Gillespie's sea-lion. Ileo-colic junction and cæcum; dried preparation. (Columbia University Museum, No. 90.)

FIG. 396.—*Phoca vitulina*, harbor seal. Ileo-colic junction and cæcum. (Columbia University Museum, No. 762.)

FIG. 397.—*Vulpes fulvus*, red fox. Ileo-colic junction and cæcum; dried preparation. (Columbia University Museum, No. 114.)

B. FISSIPEDIA.—The *Cynoidea*, including the dogs, jackals, wolves and foxes, form a well-marked central group with well-developed convoluted cæca placed laterally to the ileo-colic junction (Figs. 397-399).

FIG. 398.—*Canis familiaris*, dog. Ileo-colic junction and cæcum, Type I. (Columbia University Museum, No. 1550.)

FIG. 399.—*Canis familiaris*, dog. Ileo-colic junction and cæcum, Type II. (Columbia University Museum, No. 1551.)

FIG. 400.—*Genetta vulgaris*, genet. Ileo-colic junction and cæcum. (Columbia University Museum, No. 1625.)

FIG. 401.—*Felis concolor*, puma. Ileo-colic junction and cæcum; dried preparation. (Columbia University Museum, No. 119.)

FIG. 402.—*Felis borealis, var. rufus*, red lynx. Ileo-colic junction and cæcum; dried preparation. (Columbia University Museum, No. 177.)

FIG. 404.—*Herpestes sp.?*, ichneumon. Ileo-colic junction and cæcum; dried preparation. (Columbia University Museum, No. 120.)

FIG. 403.—*Paradoxurus typus*, paradoxure. Ileo-colic junction and cæcum; dried preparation. (Columbia University Museum, No. 112.)

FIG. 405.—*Herpestes griseus*, mongoose ichneumon. Ileo-colic junction and cæcum; dried preparation. (Columbia University Museum, No. 149.)

From this type depart on the one hand the *Ailuroidea*, including the civets, ichneumons and true cats, with the cæcum uniformly present, but short and markedly pointed, suggesting the degeneration of a formerly better developed structure (Figs. 400-406), while on the other the *Arctoidea*, including the bears, weasels and raccoons, constitute a group united by many common fundamental peculiarities of structure, among which is the entire absence of a cæcal pouch (Figs. 407-415).

FIG. 406.—*Proteles lalandii*, aard-wolf. Ileo-colic junction and cæcum. (Columbia University Museum, No. 1520.)

FIG. 407.—*Nasua rufa*, brown coati-mundi. Ileo-colic junction. (Columbia University Museum, No. 1089.)

FIG. 408.—*Nasua rufa*, brown coati-mundi. Ileo-colic junction, opened, showing pyloric-like ileo-colic valve. (Columbia University Museum, No. 1581.)

FIG. 409.—*Bassaris astuta*, raccoon-fox. Ileo-colic junction; dried preparation. (Columbia University Museum, No. 289.)

FIG. 410.—*Mustela sp.?*, marten. Ileo-colic junction; dried preparation. (Columbia University Museum, No. 199.)

FIG. 411.—*Taxidea americana*, American badger. Ileo-colic junction; dried preparation. (Columbia University Museum, No. 180.)

FIG. 412.—*Procyon lotor*, raccoon. Ileo-colic junction; dried preparation. (Columbia University Museum, No. 230.)

FIG. 413.—*Cercoleptes caudivolvulus*, kinkajou. Ileo-colic junction; dried preparation. (Columbia University Museum, No. 295.)

FIG. 414.—*Ursus americanus*, black bear. Ileo-colic junction; dried preparation. (Columbia University Museum, No. 226.)

FIG. 415.—*Ursus maritimus*, polar bear. Ileo-colic junction. (Columbia University Museum, No. 748.)

FIG. 416.—*Hyæna striata*, striped hyena. Ileo-colic junction and cæcum; dried preparation. (Columbia University Museum, No. 56.)

FIG. 417.—*Felis leo*, lion, Ileo-colic junction and cæcum. (Columbia University Museum, No. 1516.)

Among the ailuroid carnivora, the hyæna and the lion occupy an isolated position in regard to the cæcum. Both of these animals possess a well-developed long cæcal pouch with blunt extremity (Figs. 416 and 417). They probably afford examples of a persistent ancestral common type from which the remaining carnivorous forms are derived by reduction of the cæcal apparatus in conformity with the food-habits of these animals. The cæcum of both the lion and hyæna resembles very closely the pouch of the herbivorous marsupials, such as*Halmaturus* or *Didelphis* (cf. Figs. 348 and 350, p. 205).

IX. Order: Cheiroptera.

In the bats the alimentary canal is uniformly simple without cæcum and scarcely any differentiation between small and large intestine (Fig. 418).

FIG. 418.—*Pteropus medius*, Indian fruit-bat. Ileo-colon; dried preparation. (Columbia University Museum, No. 533.)

X. Order: Insectivora.

In the true Insectivora the cæcum is also absent and the alimentary canal a simple non-differentiated tube.

In certain herbivorous animals included in this group on the other hand, such as*Galeopithecus* (Fig. 419), the cæcum is present as an enormous sacculated pouch with spiral convolutions.

FIG. 419.—*Galeopithecus volans*, colugo. Ileo-colic junction, cæcum, and colon. (Columbia University Museum, No. 1844.)

XI. Order: Primates.

The cæcum is uniformly present. In certain of the Lemuroidea the terminal portion of the pouch is reduced, forming a species of appendix. A typical vermiform appendix is regularly found in man and in the anthropoid apes, orang, gibbon, chimpanzee and gorilla.

1. Suborder Lemuroidea.

In the typical lemurs the cæcum is long, frequently terminating in a pointed appendage. The proximal segment of the colon is looped and coiled, resembling the spiral colon of the Ungulates and Rodents. Fig. 420 shows the cæcum of *Nycticebus tardigradus*, the slow lemur, with the typical appendage, and Fig. 421 shows the spiral arrangement of the proximal colon immediately beyond the ileo-colic junction in the same animal. Fig. 422, taken from another specimen of the same animal shows the cæcum, appendix and spiral colon. Figs. 423, 424, 425 illustrate the structure of the parts in three other members of the group, *Lemur macaco*, *Lemur mongoz* and *Otolicnus crassicaudatus*, all showing terminal reduction of the cæcal pouch and tendency to spiral coiling of the proximal colon. In *Tarsius spectrum* (Fig. 426) the cæcum is relatively well-developed, but forms a simple pouch of uniform diameter, without terminal reduction.

FIG. 420.—*Nycticebus tardigradus*, slow lemur. Ileo-colic junction, cæcum, appendix, and colon; dorsal view. (Columbia University Museum, No. 20/1468.)

FIG. 421.—*Nycticebus tardigradus*, slow lemur. Same preparation as Fig. 420; ventral view, showing spiral coiling of proximal colon. (Columbia University Museum, No. 20/1468.)

FIG. 422.—*Nycticebus tardigradus*, slow lemur. Ileo-colic junction, cæcum, appendix, and spiral colon. (Columbia University, Study Collection.)

FIG. 423.—*Lemur macaco*, lemur. Ileo-colic junction and cæcum. (Drawn from preparation.) (Columbia University Museum, No. 1623.)

FIG. 424.—*Lemur mongoz*, lemur. Ileo-colic junction and cæcum. (Drawn from preparation.) (Columbia University Museum, No. 1473.)

FIG. 425.—*Otolicnus crassicaudatus*, galago. Ileo-colic junction and cæcum. (Drawn from preparation.) (Columbia University Museum, No. 1626.)

FIG. 426.—*Tarsius spectrum*, spectre lemur. (Drawn from preparation.) (Columbia University Museum, No. 1521.)

2. Suborder Anthropoidea.

110

1. Cynocephalus.—The baboons have a well-developed capacious cæcum. The apex of the pouch is usually blunt and rounded, or only slightly pointed. The cæcum is sacculated, conforming in structure to the rest of the large intestine. Two low vascular folds or ridges, a ventral and a dorsal, carry the ventral and dorsal cæcal branches of the ileo-colic artery. The intermediate non-vascular fold is large, frequently fused with the dorsal vascular fold (cf.p. 264).

Figs. 427-433 show the structures in *Cynocephalus sphinx, porcarius, babuin, anubis* and in *Cercopithecus pogonias, sabæus* and *campbellii.*

FIG. 427.—*Cynocephalus sphinx*, Guinea baboon. Ileo-colic junction and cæcum. (Columbia University Museum, No. 1082.)

FIG. 428.—*Cynocephalus porcarius,* Chacma baboon. Ileo-colic junction and cæcum. (Columbia University Museum, No. 1071.)

FIG. 429.—*Cynocephalus babuin,* yellow baboon; dried preparation. (Columbia University Museum, No. 89.)

FIG. 430.—*Cynocephalus anubis*, olive baboon. (Columbia University Museum, No. 51/1618.)

FIG. 431.—*Cercopithecus pogonias,* bearded monkey. Ileo-colic junction and cæcum; dried preparation. (Columbia University Museum, No. 228.)

FIG. 432.—*Cercopithecus sabæus,* green monkey. Ileo-colic junction and cæcum. (Drawn from preparation.) (Columbia University Museum, No. 746.)

FIG. 433.—*Cercopithecus campbellii,* cercopithecus monkey. Ileo-colic junction and cæcum. (Drawn from preparation.) (Columbia University Museum, No. 55/1542.)

1. Ventral ileo-cæcal vascular fold.
2. Dorsal ileo-cæcal vascular fold.
3. Intermediate ileo-cæcal non-vascular fold.

2. Macacus.—The cæcum is of large caliber, blunt, or in some forms slightly pointed at the apex, sacculated like the colon.

The two vascular folds are narrow and low, studded with epiploic appendages. The intermediate non-vascular fold is large, placed nearer to the dorsal than to the ventral vascular fold.

Figs. 434-439 show the structures in *Macacus cynomolgus, ochreatus, rhesus* and *pileatus.*

Fig. 439 is from a formaline hardened situs preparation of the abdominal viscera in *Macacus cynomolgus*, the Kra monkey.

FIG. 434.—*Macacus cynomolgus,* Macaque monkey. Ileo-colic junction and cæcum; dried preparation. (Columbia University Museum, No. 19.)

FIG. 436.—*Macacus rhesus*, rhesus monkey. Ileo-colic junction and cæcum. (Columbia University Museum, No. 1126.)

FIG. 435.—

111

Macacus ochreatus, ashy-black macaque. Ileo-colic junction and cæcum; dried preparation. (Columbia University Museum, No. 11.)

FIG. 438.—*Macacus sinicus,* bonnet macaque. Ileo-colic junction and cæcum. (Columbia University Museum, No. 1072.)

FIG. 437.—*Macacus pileatus,* macaque. Ileo-colic junction and cæcum. (Columbia University Museum, No. 719.)

FIG. 439.—*Macacus cynomolgus,* kra monkey. Abdominal viscera, hardened *in situ.* (Columbia University Museum, No. 1801.)

B. ARCTOPITHECINI.

The marmosets have a long crescentic-shaped cæcum, turning the concavity of the curve upwards and to the left, terminating in a blunt point.

Typical forms are shown in Fig. 440, *Hapale jacchus,* Fig. 441, *Midas ursulus,* and Fig. 442, *Midas geoffrei.*

FIG. 440.—*Hapule jacchus,* common marmoset. Ileo-colic junction and cæcum. (Columbia University Museum, No. 975.)

FIG. 441.—*Midas ursulus,* negro tamarin. Ileo-colic junction and cæcum; dried preparation. (Columbia University Museum, No. 235.)

FIG. 442.—*Midas geoffrei,* Geoffrey's marmoset. Ileo-colic junction and cæcum; dried preparation. (Columbia University Museum, No. 197.)

C. CEBIDÆ.

1. Ateles and other howlers have a large cæcum, crescentic in shape, narrowed at the apex, separated from the colon by a sharp and deep constriction, opposite the wedge-shaped ileo-colic junction.

The ileo-cæcal folds are well-developed and symmetrical, two equal vascular folds, and a free intermediate non-vascular reduplication.

Types: *Ateles ater* (Figs. 443-445), *Chrysothrix sciureus* (Fig. 447) and *Nyctipithecus commersonii* (Fig. 446). In *Mycetes* (Figs. 448-450) the pouch is shorter, less curved, with a slight reduction toward the less distinctly pointed apex.

FIG. 443.—*Ateles ater,* black-faced coaita. Ileo-colic junction and cæcum; dried preparation. (Columbia University Museum, No. 240.)

FIG. 444.—*Ateles ater,* black-faced coaita. Ileo-colic junction and cæcum, with ileo-cæcal folds. (Columbia University Museum, No. 720.)

FIG. 445.—*Ateles ater,* black-faced coaita. Ileo-colic junction and cæcum, with ileo-cæcal folds. (Drawn from preparation.) (Columbia University Museum, No. 300.)

1. Ventral vascular ileo-cæcal fold.
2. Intermediate non-vascular ileo-cæcal fold.
3. Dorsal vascular ileo-cæcal fold.

FIG. 446.—*Nyctipithecus commersonii,* Vitœ monkey. Ileo-colic junction and cæcum; dried preparation. (Columbia University Museum, No. 238.)

FIG. 447.—*Chrysothrix sciureus,* Viti monkey. Ileo-colic junction and cæcum. (Columbia University

FIG. 448.—*Mycetes cavaya,* black howler. Ileo-colic junction and cæcum. (Columbia University Museum, No. 1136.)

FIG. 449.—*Mycetes fuscus*, brown howler. Ileo-colic junction and cæcum, with ileo-cæcal folds; ventral view. (Columbia University Museum, No. 674.)

1. Ventral vascular ileo-cæcal fold.
3. Intermediate non-vascular ileo-cæcal fold.

FIG. 450.—Drawn from the same preparation as Fig. 449; dorsal view.

2. Dorsal vascular ileo-cæcal fold.
3. Intermediate non-vascular ileo-cæcal fold.

2. Lagothrix.—The cæcum is very capacious and long, bent at a sharp angle upwards and to the left toward the ileo-colic junction.

Type: *Lagothrix humboldtii* (Fig. 451).

FIG. 451.—*Lagothrix humboldtii*, Humboldt's lagothrix. Ileo-colic junction and cæcum. (Columbia University Museum, No. 1511.)

3. Pithecia.—The cæcum resembles in general the type presented by *Ateles*, but is less curved and less reduced and pointed at the termination.

Type: *Pithecia satanas* (Fig. 452).

FIG. 452.—*Pithecia satanas*, black saki monkey. Ileo-colic junction and cæcum. (Columbia University Museum, No. 641.)

In general the Arctopithecini and *Ateles*, *Mycetes*, *Lagothrix* and *Pithecia* among the Cebidæ form a group containing a series of cæcal transition types which lead up to the anthropomorphous type, illustrating the following conditions:

(*a*) The inherent crescentic curve of the cæcum, with the concavity directed toward the left, and carrying the apex of the pouch upward toward the lower border of the ileum and the ileo-colic junction. (*Hapalidæ, Ateles, Lagothrix.*)

(*b*) The reduction in caliber of the terminal part, foreshadowing by the pointed and narrow extremity of the pouch the appearance of the appendix in the anthropomorphous group. (*Hapalidæ, Ateles.*)

(*c*) The constriction at the level of the ileo-cæcal junction, with the corresponding well-marked differentiation between cæcum and colon in the interior. (*Ateles.*)

(*d*) The sharp bend in the pouch as it makes its turn upward and to the left, repeated in certain types of adult human cæca (cf. p. 247). (*Lagothrix.*)

(*e*) *Pithecia* forms a transitive type between the blunt sacculated cæca of the Cynomorpha and the curved pointed pouches of the Cebidæ, partaking of the characters of both.

(*f*) The same character is seen in the cæcum of *Mycetes fuscus* the brown howler monkey (Figs. 449 and 450).

4. Cebinæ.—In the typical genus *Cebus* the cæcum is placed laterad to the small intestine which is in direct linear continuity with the colon. The pouch is slightly convoluted toward its termination, resembling in this respect and in its position relative to the lumen of the intestinal canal, the disposition of the parts in the cynoid carnivora. Figs. 453 and 454 show the structures in two typical species, *Cebus monachus* and *C. leucophæus*.

FIG. 453.—*Cebus monachus*, capuchin monkey. Ileo-colic junction and cæcum; dried preparation. (Columbia University Museum, No. 26.)

FIG. 454.—*Cebus leucophæus*, capuchin monkey. Ileo-colic junction and cæcum. (Columbia University Museum, No. 1467.)

D. ANTHROPOMORPHA.

The cæcum is large, sacculated, provided uniformly with a vermiform appendix.

The pouch of the four anthropoid apes agrees in curve, direction, implantation of the appendix and the general arrangement of the vascular and peritoneal folds with the structure in the human subject.

1. Hylobates hoolock, Gibbon.—Figs. 455 and 456 represent respectively the ileo-cæcum of this animal in the ventral view, and from the left side with the ileum turned forward. The cæcum is a globular rounded pouch of nearly uniform diameter, only slightly enlarged to the right of the root of the appendix which arises from its lowest part and is pendent.

FIG. 455.—*Hylobates hoolock*, hoolock gibbon. Ileo-colic junction and cæcum; ventral view. (Drawn from Columbia University Museum preparation No. 1530.)

FIG. 456.—Drawn from same preparation as Fig. 455; view from left side, showing formation of posterior ileo-cæcal fossa.

FIG. 457.—*Gorilla savagei*, gorilla. Ileo-colic junction and cæcum, with ileo-cæcal folds. (Drawn from Columbia University Museum preparation No. 1543.)

(For arrangement of the ileo-cæcal folds and fossæ in this form see p. 269.)

2. Gorilla savagei, Gorilla (Fig. 457).—The cæcum is large, distinctly sacculated, presenting a decided curve with the concavity directed toward the left. The appendix is implanted at the center of the blunt apex of the pouch, the cæcal sacculations on each side of the root of the appendix being of nearly equal size (folds and fossæ, cf. p. 269).

FIG. 458.—*Simia satyrus*, orang. Cæcum and ileo-colic junction; ventral view. (Drawn from Columbia University Museum preparation No. 716.) 1. Appendix. 2. Ventral vascular fold.

FIG. 459.—*Simia satyrus*, orang. Cæcum and ileo-colic junction; dorsal view. (Drawn from Columbia University Museum preparation No. 716). 1. Appendix. 2. Intermediate non-vascular fold.

3. Simia satyrus, Orang-outang.—Figs. 458 and 459 represent respectively the ventral and dorsal views of the cæcum and ileo-colon in a nearly adult male specimen of orang, about 4½ feet high.

The cæcum is funnel-shaped, gradually narrowing to the origin of the appendix from its apex, which is carried upwards to the left by the well-marked crescentic curve of the pouch. The sweep of the funnel to the left and upwards is characterized by the curved course of the ventral longitudinal muscular band (Fig. 458), whose fibers spread out over a surface 3 cm. wide. The apex is thus placed behind the terminal ileum close to its entrance into the large intestine.

At the level of the upper margin of the ileo-colic junction the narrow pointed termination of the cæcum passes gradually into the beginning of the appendix (Fig. 459).

The appendix measures along its free border 22.6 cm. It follows the direction of the cæcal curve for 2.7 cm., at which point it appears somewhat constricted and takes an abrupt bend downwards for 4.3 cm.; curving again upwards for 7.5 cm., it turns downward a second time for 5.4 cm. and terminates in a hook-like extremity 2.7 cm. long (Fig. 459).

FIG. 460.—*Troglodytes niger*, chimpanzee. Ileo-colic junction and cæcum; ventral view. (Drawn from Columbia University Museum preparation No. 675.) 1. Appendix. 2. Intermediate non-vascular ileo-cæcal fold. 3. Colon.

FIG. 461.—*Troglodytes niger*, chimpanzee. Dorsal view. (Drawn from Columbia University Museum preparation No. 675.) 1. Appendix. 2. Intermediate non-vascular ileo-cæcal fold. 3. Dorsal vascular fold.

4. Chimpanzee, Troglodytes niger.—Figs. 460 and 461 represent the ventral and dorsal view respectively of the cæcum and ileo-colon in a young specimen.

The cæcum is curved to the left and the lowest point of the pouch is formed by the right lateral and ventral wall of the gut, but the extreme crescentic bend which carries the origin of the appendix up and to the left behind the ileo-colic junction is not yet developed in the young animal; on the other hand this character of the cæcum is typically apparent in Figs. 462 and 463, taken from an adult individual of the same species.

FIG. 462.—*Troglodytes niger*, chimpanzee. Ileo-colic junction and cæcum; ventral view. (Drawn from Columbia University Museum preparation No. 1083.) 1.

FIG. 463.—*Troglodytes niger*, chimpanzee. Ileo-colic junction and cæcum; dorsal view. (Drawn from Columbia University Museum preparation No. 1083.) 1. Appendix.

Ventral vascular ileo-cæcal fold.

FIG. 464.—*Troglodytes niger*, chimpanzee. Ileo-colic junction and cæcum. (Drawn from Columbia University Museum preparation No. 1525.)

This extreme curve is well seen in the ventral view in Figs. 462 and 464, the latter taken from a large adult specimen. Seen from behind in Fig. 463 the sharp bend or kink in the lumen of the cæcal pouch produced by this curve is striking and resembles the arrangement of certain types of adult human cæca (p. 247).

II. PHYLOGENY OF THE TYPES OF ILEO-COLIC JUNCTION AND CÆCUM IN THE VERTEBRATE SERIES.

The segments of the alimentary canal illustrate very clearly the adaptation of structure to function. Diversity of kind and quantity of food habitually taken and variations in the rapidity of tissue metabolism produce marked morphological modifications in different forms. This is more especially the case with the junction of the mid- and hindgut, the site of development of the cæcal apparatus and of structural alterations of the large intestine possessing a similar physiological significance. No other portion of the visceral tract, with the possible exception of the stomach, illustrates more completely the result of physiological demand on the development of anatomical structure and the morphological possibilities of departure, progressive and retrograde, from a common primitive type in accordance with varying conditions of alimentation.

In coördinating, from the morphological standpoint, the structural differences encountered in this segment of the alimentary canal, two facts become apparent.

1. In the first place the serial study of the ileo-colic junction, as we can briefly define the region in question by borrowing the terminology of anthropotomy, reveals a limited number of principal structural types from which by successive gradations the vast variety of individual forms may be derived.

FIG. 465.—Schematic table of the vertebrate types of ileo-colic junction.

(In the schematic Fig. 465 the fundamental types and their derivatives are indicated. In the following the individual forms illustrating these types are referred to this schema in brackets.)

2. The observer will be impressed by the fact that representatives of all the main types of ileo-colic junction are found within a very limited zoölogical range, as within the confines of a single order. Examples of this are furnished by the Marsupialia and, to a lesser extent, by the Edentata. The members of these zoölogical groups, while united by certain common anatomical characters, such as the reproductive system and dentition, differ widely in habit and in the kind and quantity of the food normally taken. These differences in the method of nutrition have impressed their influence on the structure of the alimentary canal and have led to the evolution of varying and divergent types of ileo-colic junction. The study of this segment of the intestinal tract can therefore elucidate the mutual relationship of the vertebrate groups only to a limited degree and in special cases. On the other hand, it renders very clear the fundamental structural ground-plan common to all vertebrates and accentuates the specialized modifications of this plan which develop in response to the physiological environment. Moreover, such a review serves to reveal the significance of rudimentary and vestigial structures, such as the human vermiform appendix and the serous and vascular folds connected with the same. Throughout the entire vertebrate series the alimentary canal is found to respond with great readiness in its structure to varying grades of functional demand. This fact becomes still more apparent if the inquiry is not limited strictly to the region of the ileo-colic junction but takes into account likewise the structural modifications of similar physiological significance in other segments of the alimentary tract.

A cæcal pouch or diverticulum in some form at the junction of mid- and hindgut is a very common and widely distributed mammalian character. The activity of the tissue-changes in warm-blooded animals, and the consequent necessity for a rapid and complete digestive process, account for the structural modifications of the alimentary tract so commonly encountered among these forms. On the other hand, in the lower cold-blooded vertebrates, notably in fishes and amphibians, the metabolism is slow and the alimentary canal usually simple.

Specifically, the cæcum appears as a pouch or diverticulum in which food-substances, already partially digested and mixed with the secretions of the small intestine, are retained until their elaboration is completed and the nutritive value of the food ingested is secured for the organism. Consequently the most complicated and highly developed cæcal apparatus is found among mammalia in the Herbivora, such as the Ungulates and Rodents, whose food contains a comparatively small amount of nutriment in ratio to its bulk, and hence requires considerable elaboration before absorption. On the other hand the cæcum appears as a reduced or even rudimentary organ, or defaults entirely, in Carnivora whose food is concentrated and easily assimilated, containing only a small amount of non-nutritive material.

The function of the cæcal apparatus may be defined as follows:

FIG. 466.—*Squalus acanthius*, dog-fish. Alimentary tract, spleen, pancreas. (Drawn from Columbia University Museum preparation No. 1405.)

1. It provides space for the retention of partly digested substances, and of such as are difficult of digestion, mixed with thesecretions of the preceding intestinal segment, until the digestive elaboration is completed.

2. It increases the intestinal mucous surface for absorption, and may develop, in certain cases, special localized areas of lymphoid tissue.

These two functional characters may be shared by other segments of the intestinal tract, which undergo corresponding structural modifications. It is only necessary to refer in this connection to the extreme morphological variations encountered in the stomach. The intestinal canal proper, however, in many instances exhibits structural peculiarities which possess the functional significance of the cæcal apparatus. Thus the projection into the lumen of the canal of a series of mucous folds, or the development of a continuous spiral mucous valve, evidently serves the double purpose of prolonging the period during which the intestinal contents are retained, and of increasing the intestinal mucous surface for absorption.

FIG. 467.—*Galeus canis*, dog-shark. Alimentary tract opened, showing spiral intestinal valve. (Drawn from Columbia University Museum preparation No. 1429.)

FIG. 468.—*Ceratodus forsteri*, Australian lung-fish. Intestinal canal with spiral valve. (Columbia University Museum, No. 1645.)

This spiral mucous fold is encountered in the straight intestinal canal of the Cyclostomata (Fig. 465, *IV*, 1, and Fig. 310), Selachians (Figs. 466 and 467) and Dipnœans (Fig. 468). Phylogenetically it is a very old structure, for evidences of its existence are found in the fossil remains of some Elasmobranchs. In the Ostrich (Fig. 341) the enormously developed cæca possess the same spiral mucous fold in the interior. The direct combination of the cæcum and spiral fold is again seen in certain mammalia, as in *Lepus* (Fig. 387). In some Ophidians the same physiological purpose is served by the manner in which the convolutions of the long intestine are bound together by a subperitoneal arachnoid membrane. The lumen of the canal is thus made to assume a spiral course (Figs. 331 and 469). The mucous folds of the human intestine, both the valvulæ conniventes and the crescentic folds of the large intestine, represent the same spiral valve, perhaps modified and influenced by the erect posture of man (Figs. 470-475).

FIG. 470.—Human small intestine, opened to show valvulæ conniventes. (Columbia University Museum, No. 1841.)

FIG. 469.—*Python molurus*, Indian python. Mid-gut, distended and fenestrated to show spiral course of lumen. (Columbia University Museum, No. 725.)

FIG. 472.—Human large intestine, opened and in section, showing colic plicæ. (Columbia University Museum, No. 1847.)

FIG. 471.—Human large intestine, showing colic tænia and plica. (Columbia University Museum, No. 1848.)

FIG. 473.—*Cynocephalus*

FIG. 474.—Comparison of portion of

anubis, olive baboon. Large intestine, with cross-section showing colic tænia and plicæ. (Columbia University Museum, No. 26/1168.)

human transverse colon with distal segment of rabbit's large intestine, showing same arrangement of longitudinal muscular bands (colic tænia) and colic sacculations. (Columbia University Museum, No. 1589.)

FIG. 475.—*Felis leo*, lion. Large intestine, with transverse section, showing smooth carnivore lumen, without sacculations or plicæ. (Columbia University Museum, No. 1600.)

FIG. 476.—Pyloric cæca of *Gadus callarias*, codfish. (Columbia University Museum, No. 1825.)

A. Bound together by connective tissue and blood-vessels.

B. Dissected to show confluence of cæca to form a smaller number of terminal tubes of larger calibre entering the intestine.

FIG. 477.—Alimentary canal of *Accipenser sturio*, sturgeon. Numerous pyloric cæca are bound together to form a gland-like organ.

In the smaller upper figure on the left the stomach, mid-gut, and pyloric cæca are seen in section, showing the lumen of the latter and their openings into the mid-gut.

The lower left-hand figure shows the mid- and end-gut in section, the latter provided with a spiral mucous valve. (Columbia University Museum, Nos. 1826, 1827, and 1828.)

A second modification of the intestinal canal, suggesting the same physiological interpretation as the ileo-colic cæcum, is presented by the so-called pyloric cæca or appendices of many Teleosts and Ganoids already referred to (p. 119). While these structures in some forms very probably have assumed a secretory function (Figs. 476 and 477), they evidently act in others as diverticula in which material undergoing digestion is retained, while they increase at the same time the intestinal mucous secretory and absorbing surface (Figs. 478 and 479). They thus correspond physiologically to the ileo-colic cæcum. In this connection it is interesting to note that in Ganoids, which possess both the pyloric appendices and the spiral valve, the two structures develop in inverse ratio to each other, indicating their functional identity. In the serial review of the structure and significance of the vertebrate cæcum and ileo-colic junction these functionally allied modifications of other segments of the intestinal canal deserve notice.

The study of the vertebrate ileo-colic junction proper begins both ontogenetically and phylogenetically with the consideration of the primitive type in which the alimentary tube is not differentiated into successive segments and in which consequently no distinction between mid- and hindgut is found (Fig. 465). An example of this primitive condition is presented by the Cyclostomata, in whom the alimentary canal traverses the cœlom cavity as a straight non-differentiated cylindrical tube. Fig. 310 shows the alimentary canal of the Lamprey, *Petromyzon marinus*, and it will be observed that the intestine is provided with the spiral mucous fold above mentioned.

From this fundamental type the following main groups are to be derived:

FIG. 478.—Stomach, duodenum, and pyloric cæca of *Lophius piscatorius*, angler. (Columbia University Museum, No. 1824.)

FIG. 479.—*Pleuronectes maculatus*, window-pane. Stomach and mid-gut with pyloric cæca and hepatic duct. (Columbia University Museum, No. 1432.)

I. Symmetrical Form of Ileo-colic Junction. Mid- and Endgut in Direct Linear Continuity. (Fig. 465, I.)

1. *Ileo-colic junction marked externally by an annular constriction, corresponding to a ring-valve with central circular opening in the interior* (Fig. 465, I, 1).

This form is encountered in many Teleosts. The projecting annular mucous fold resembles the pyloro-duodenal valve.

Figs. 311-315 illustrate the structures in representative Teleosts.

Among the higher forms this type of ileo-colic junction is encountered in the simple alimentary canal of many Amphibians (Figs. 318-320). Among Reptiles it is found in certain lizards, as in *Heloderma suspectum*, the gila monster (Fig. 322). This animal lives almost entirely upon bird's eggs, and its simple and reduced ileo-colic junction contrasts strongly with the highly developed and complicated cæcal apparatus of the phytophagous lizards, as *Iguana* (Figs. 326-330), affording one of the most striking illustrations of the effect which the character of the food habitually taken has on the structure of the alimentary canal in forms otherwise closely allied.

The same type of ileo-colic junction, as a reduction form, occurs in the arctoid group of Carnivora among Mammalia (cf. p. 212).

2. *Differentiation in caliber of large and small intestine. Funnel-shaped ileo-colic transition.*

This type, compared with the preceding, is characterized (Fig. 465, *I*, 2) by the greatly increased caliber of the large intestine, resulting in a funnel-shaped transition between mid- and hindgut, the small intestine continuing into the colon at the apex of the funnel.

Examples of this type are presented by several Edentates, *Myrmecophaga jubata*, the great ant-eater (Fig. 356), and *Cholœpus didactylus*, the two-toed sloth (Fig. 357).

3. *Abrupt demarcation of small and large intestine with caliber differentiation* (Fig. 465, *I*, 3).

The small intestine is still central at the ileo-colic junction, *i. e.*, the axis of its lumen is continuous with the central axis of the colic lumen. In place of the gradual funnel-shaped transition of the preceding type the demarcation is abrupt.

An example of this form is furnished by another Edentate, *Tatusia peba*, the nine-banded armadillo (Fig. 358).

Among reptiles a similar well-marked ileo-colic transition is encountered in *Alligator mississippiensis* (Fig. 321).

4. *Colic pouch prolonged back on each side of the ileo-colic junction, producing symmetrical colic cæca* (Fig. 465, *I*, 4).

A growth of the colic tube cephalad, on each side of the junction with the midgut, leads to the formation of this type, characterized by the presence of two symmetrical globular cæcal pouches. In its simplest form this condition is illustrated by the double colic cæca of another armadillo, *Dasypus sexcinctus* (Fig. 359).

The bifid cæcal apparatus of the American manatee (Fig. 366) belongs to the same group.

5. *Cæcal pouches of the birds* (Fig. 465, *I*, 5).—A continuation of the backward extension of the bilateral colic pouches leads to the production of the typical double avian cæca in a greater or lesser degree of development. Frequently the cæca differentiate more completely from the colon, appearing as pouches of varying capacity joined to the large intestine by a narrower neck.

Figs. 334-341 show the well-developed pouches as they appear in representative avian types, while Fig. 333 illustrates the reduction of the cæcal apparatus encountered in many carnivorous birds.

6. Among mammalia *Cyclothurus didactylus* (Fig. 360), the little ant-eater, furnishes an example of double symmetrical globular cæca, connected with the colon by a narrow neck (Fig. 465, *I*, 6). Reference to the schema given in Fig. 465 will show that the types heretofore examined all have the following common character:

They appear derived from the primitive type by a differentiation in the caliber of the gut and by the gradual development of *symmetrical bilateral* cæcal pouches, resulting in central median implantation of the small intestine and its direct continuity with the colon.

II. Asymmetrical Development of a Single Cæcal Pouch, Lateral to the Ileocolic Junction, Mid- and Endgut Preserving Their Linear Continuity. (Fig. 465, II.)

In the second general group the symmetry of the ileo-colic junction is disturbed. The following types are encountered, forming a series of successive stages:

1. The increase in the caliber of the large intestine is chiefly marked along the border opposite to the mesenteric attachment, resulting in a greater degree of convexity in this part of the intestinal wall (Fig. 465, *II*, 1). Among Reptilia this condition is found in the ileo-colic junction of some of the pond-turtles, as *Pseudemys elegans* (Fig. 323), while a mammalian example is furnished by the three-toed sloth, *Arctopithecus marmoratus* (Fig. 363).

2. An increase of this lateral extension of the colon leads to the formation of a single lateral cæcal pouch (Fig. 465, *II*, 2) such as is seen in another Edentate, *Tamandua*

bivittata (Fig. 364), among Mammalia, and in certain Ophidians among Reptiles, as in the *Anaconda*(Figs. 331 and 332).

3. Prolongation of the pouch and reduction in caliber lead to the formation of the slender lateral cæcum found in all the Monotremes (Figs. 345-347, Fig. 465, *I*, 3). In its general appearance the cæcum of these singular animals bears a close resemblance to the cæcal pouches of many birds.

4. Direct continuity of small and large intestine, with lateral colic cæcum, extending along the convex free border of the terminal ileum and slightly convoluted at the extremity (Fig. 465, *II*, 4), characterizes the entire group of the *Cebidæ* among the new-world monkeys. The cæcum in these animals is a comparatively long pouch, nearly equalling in caliber the remainder of the intestine, occupying a distinctly *lateral* position, with the terminal portion rounded and slightly recurved (Figs. 453 and 454).

5. The *Cynoid group* of Carnivora, including the dogs, wolves, jackals and foxes, presents a similar relative position of small and large intestine and cæcum (Fig. 465, *II*, 5). The cæcum, compared with that of *Cebus*, is longer and more highly convoluted (Fig. 397). Variations encountered in certain forms indicate reversions to a more primitive type. ThusFig. 398 shows the usual form in the dog, while Fig. 399 exhibits an occasional type in the same animal. The cæcum here is less twisted and indicates the probable derivation of the more commonly encountered type.

III. Rectangular Ileo-colic Junction with Direct Linear Continuity of Cæcum and Colon. (Fig. 465, III.)

The third general group, to which the large majority of Mammalia belong, is characterized in its typical form by a right-angled entrance of ileum into large intestine and by the direct caudal prolongation of the colon into a cæcal pouch of nearly uniform caliber with globular termination. The axes of the small and large intestine are not in the same line as in the two former groups, but are placed nearly at right angles to each other. With this change in the direction of the main intestinal segments the cæcum ceases to be a lateral appendage to the canal and appears as a caudal prolongation of the colon beyond the ileo-colic junction (Fig. 465, *III*). The type-form of this group is encountered among the herbivorous Marsupialia, such as the kangaroos and opossums. Fig. 350 shows the ileo-colic junction and cæcum in the rock wallaby, *Halmaturus derbyanus*, and Fig. 348 the same structures in our common opossum, *Didelphis virginiana*. The majority of the remaining mammalian forms depend upon modifications of this type, either in the direction of reduction of the cæcal apparatus, or of increased development with concomitant structural changes of similar physiological import in the proximal portion of the colon.

The following subdivisions of the general group may be established.

A. 1. The cæcum is long, markedly curved or uncinate, with the crescentic medial margin turned toward the free border of the terminal ileum. The entire pouch usually diminishes gradually in caliber to its termination (Fig. 465, *III*, *A*, 1). This type is encountered in a large group of new-world monkeys, including the marmosets and howlers.

Fig. 440 shows the structures in *Hapale jacchus*, one of the marmosets, and Fig. 443illustrates the typical cæcum of this form in *Ateles ater*, the black-handed spider monkey.

2. The cæcum and appendix of man and of the anthropoid apes can be regarded as a reduction form of this type (Fig. 465, *III*, *A*, 2). Arrest of development of the terminal portion converts the distal segment of the cæcal pouch into an appendix whose relation to the apex of the funnel-shaped proximal segment or cæcum proper is seen in its pure form in the human embryo (Figs. 512 and 525). With the further development of the cæcum the sharper demarcation between it and the appendix results (Figs. 517 and 518). The displacement of the root of the appendix cephalad and to the left, toward the lower margin of the ileo-colic junction, as it is usually seen in adults, is due to the relatively greater growth of the right terminal sacculation of the cæcum compared with the left (cf. types of cæca, p. 248). Throughout these changes the initial crescentic curve of the cæcum, turning its concavity upwards and to the left, can be recognized by tracing the course of the longitudinal colic muscular bands. The cæca and appendices of the anthropoid apes present the same characters. The structures in the orang, chimpanzee, gorilla and gibbon are shown in Figs. 455-464.

B. The Æluroid and Arctoid groups of the Carnivora and the Pinnipedia constitute a very complete and instructive series illustrating the gradual reduction of the cæcum from the capacious pouch of the primitive type and its final complete elimination from the organism (Fig. 465, *III*, *B*).

In *Hyæna* (Fig. 416), the large cæcum with undiminished caliber of the terminal portion persists in its full development, as seen in the Marsupials furnishing the fundamental type (Fig. 465, *III*). The same type of cæcum is found in the lion (Fig. 417), the only true cat in which the cæcal apparatus has not undergone extensive reduction. Phylogenetically the presence of a capacious and uniform cæcal pouch in these two animals is exceedingly important and indicates that this type of cæcum represents the ancestral form common to the æluroid carnivore group, which, in the remaining living representatives, has become reduced in response to the influence which the character of the food has on the structure of this portion of the intestinal canal. The two instances of persistence of the primal type are all the more important as exceptions to the rule which is otherwise universal throughout the group.

1. The first example of this reduction (Fig. 465, *III*, *B*, 1) is encountered in the Aard-Wolf,*Proteles lalandii*, a near relative of hyæna (Fig. 406). The cæcum in this animal is considerably shortened, although still of fairly large and uniform caliber.

A similar type of cæcal reduction is encountered in the Pinnipede Carnivora. Fig. 396 shows the ileo-colic junction and the short blunt cæcum of the harbor seal, *Phoca vitulina*.

2. The cæcum of the typical Felidæ, other than the lion, is short and the terminal portion much reduced in caliber, constituting in many forms a species of pointed rudimentary appendix (Fig. 465, *III*, *B*, 2). Fig. 401 represents the typical feline cæcum as seen in the puma, *Felis concolor*. Among the smaller Æluroid Carnivora related to the true cats, as the civets and ichneumons, the terminal reduction of the short cæcum is still more marked, as seen for example in *Herpestes griseus* (Figs. 404 and 405).

3. In the Arctoid group of Carnivora (Fig. 465, *III*, *B*, 3 and 4) the reduction of the cæcal apparatus has been carried to the complete elimination of the pouch, restoring the primitive type of a straight intestinal tube without diverticulum as encountered above in some of the Edentates (Figs. 356 and 357).

In some forms allied to the true bears, such as *Procyon*, *Bassaris*, *Cercoleptes*, *Taxidea* and*Nasua*, the ileo-colic junction is marked externally by a slight constriction and internally by the projection of an annular pylorus-like valve (Figs. 407-409). The transition from the thin-walled ileum to the thick muscular walls of the large intestine is abrupt. The latter is very short and usually increases in caliber as it approaches the anal orifice. The mucosa of the terminal ileum presents very commonly one or two large oval areas of agminated follicles near the ileo-colic junction. The mucous membrane of the large intestine is thrown into prominent longitudinal folds. Fig. 408 shows the intestine of the brown coati, *Nasua rufa*, opened on each side of the ileo-colic transition.

In some of the Arctoidea, as *Procyon* and *Nasua*, the beginning of the colon just beyond the ileo-colic valve is bowed out opposite the mesenteric border indicating the original site of the eliminated cæcum, and recalling the arrangement of the intestine encountered above in*Arctopithecus* among the Edentates (Figs. 363, 407, 412, and 465, *III*, *B*, 3). Moreover, in the same forms rudimentary vascular and serous folds around the ileo-colic junction, corresponding to similar structures found in connection with a well-developed cæcal apparatus in other mammalia, point to the former existence of a cæcum.

4. In the typical Ursidæ even these remnants and traces of a cæcal pouch have disappeared and the intestinal canal preserves a uniform caliber, without any differentiation of large and small intestine (Figs. 414 and 415, Fig. 465, *III*, *B*, 4).

C. The last subdivision of the third main group contains forms in which the large uniform pouch of the primal type appears moderately reduced in length and sacculated, terminating either in a blunt extremity or carrying a distal constricted and rudimentary segment as an appendage.

1. The first of these types is encountered in the Old World cynomorphous monkeys. In all of these animals the cæcal pouch is wide but comparatively short, of nearly uniform caliber and sacculated like the rest of the colon, of which it forms the direct caudal

continuation (Fig. 465, *III, C,* 1). The terminal portion of the pouch is usually blunt, globular and rounded (Figs. 428, 430 and 431), in a comparatively small number of forms slightly pointed (Figs. 427 and 437).

2. In the second group the terminal reduced portion persists either as a fairly distinct appendage, or in the form of a tapering pointed extremity into which the cæcal pouch proper is continued (Fig. 465, *III, C,* 2). This type is encountered in certain non-ruminant Ungulates. An example of the first condition is furnished by the cæcal apparatus of the peccary (*Dicotyles torquatus*) (Fig. 370), while the structures in *Tapirus americanus* (Fig. 377) illustrate the second form.

IV. Cæcal Apparatus Combined with Structural Modifications of the Proximal Colon of Similar Physiological Significance. (Fig. 465, IV.)

The fourth general mammalian group comprises forms in which the cæcal pouch is large, with or without terminal appendage, while in addition the large intestine develops structural modifications which possess the general functional significance of the cæcal apparatus. This highly developed and complicated structure of the alimentary canal indicates that the habitual food of these animals is bulky and difficult of digestion. Accordingly we find the group composed in main of the majority of the Ungulates and Rodents (with the exception of *Myoxus*), forms in which the diet under natural conditions is purely herbivorous. Other mammalian orders, however, also furnish representatives of this type of cæcal apparatus, the conditions as regards character and quantity of food habitually taken corresponding to those encountered among the Ungulates and Rodents. Thus the *Phalangers* among Marsupials (Fig. 352), *Galeopithecus* (Fig. 419) as an exceptional form among the Insectivora, and certain lemurs among Primates (Figs. 420-425) present examples of a highly developed and specialized type of cæcal apparatus.

The intestinal tract of these forms must therefore be considered from two points of view:

    I. The cæcum proper.

    II. The analogous structural modifications of the proximal segment of the colon.

I. CÆCUM PROPER.

The pouch of the Ungulates and Rodents, taking these forms as the typical representatives of the entire group, is usually of very large size compared with the rest of the alimentary canal. Two types are found:

1. Large capacious smooth cæcal pouch of uniform caliber (Fig. 465, *IV,* 2). This form is met with in the Muridæ among Rodents and is illustrated in Fig. 393 showing the cæcum of *Mus decumanus*, var. *albinus*, the white rat. Fig. 392 represents the entire alimentary canal of the meadow mouse, *Arvicola pennsylvanicus*, and indicates the proportion which the cæcal apparatus bears to the remainder of the intestinal tract. The typical cæcum of the Ungulates is shown in Fig. 371, taken from *Capra ægagrus*, the bezoar goat, and in Fig. 372, taken from a preparation of *Boselaphus tragocamelus*, the Nilghai.

2. The cæcal pouch is large, markedly crescentic in shape, sacculated, or provided in the interior with a more or less complete spiral valve, and reduced in caliber in the terminal segment, forming at times a pointed appendix (Fig. 465, *IV,* 3). This form is encountered typically among certain Rodents, as in *Castor fiber*, the beaver (Figs. 381 and 382), and *Erethizon dorsatus*, the Canadian porcupine (Figs. 383 and 384), but is not confined to this order. Thus cæca of very similar structure are found among the Marsupials, as in *Phascolarctos* and *Cuscus* (Fig. 352). In some of these forms the terminal reduction of the cæcum is very marked, resulting in a long narrow segment of the pouch tapering to a sharp point. It is significant to note in this connection that in one member of the marsupial order, the wombat (*Phascolomys*), this tendency to terminal reduction of the pouch has led to the development of a cæcum and appendix identical in structure and arrangement with the corresponding parts of man and the anthropoid apes (Fig. 354). This is merely another illustration of the fact, evidenced throughout the entire vertebrate series, that a primal type-form of cæcal apparatus, in responding to the conditions which influence the development of structural modifications, will produce identical specific types in animals otherwise widely separated in the zoölogical series.

Thus again the form of cæcum under discussion, found in many Rodents and certain Marsupials, is encountered in the only Insectivore possessing a cæcum (*Galeopithecus*) (Fig. 419), and in several *Lemuroidea* among Primates (Figs. 420-425).

II. Structural Modifications of the Proximal Segment of the Colon Analogous in Their Functional Significance to the Cæcal Apparatus.

In these forms, in addition to the cæcal apparatus proper, certain accessory structural modifications of the adjacent large intestine are developed which possess the physiological significance of the cæcal apparatus in general, since they serve to increase the extent of the intestinal mucous surface and to prolong the period during which the contents of the canal are retained for elaboration and absorption. These modifications, which appear most fully developed in certain Rodents and Ungulates, are of two kinds.

1. The development of the colic mucous membrane in the form of a projecting fold or valve usually surrounding the lumen spirally (Fig. 465, *IV*, 1). The significance and phylogeny of this spiral fold has been considered above (cf. p. 193). Functionally this reduplication must be regarded as in general equivalent to the cæcal apparatus proper, in producing an increased surface for secretion and absorption and in retarding the movement of intestinal contents. The cæcal pouch evidently acts as a reservoir in which partly digested substances, mixed with the secretions of the small intestine, are retained while the slow processes of digestion and absorption, already inaugurated in the antecedent segment of the canal, are completed. It is reasonable to suppose that the system of projecting mucous folds and reduplications encountered in the colon beyond the cæcum have a similar physiological import. Moreover, in certain forms the cæcum itself is provided with a similar spiral mucous fold, as in the instances already mentioned of *Lepus* among mammalia (Fig. 381) and of the Ostrich among birds (Fig. 341). We have seen above (cf. p. 193) that the spiral intestinal valve is encountered very early in the vertebrate series, in forms in which the alimentary canal is but slightly, or not at all differentiated, short and straight in its course. In these forms the evident purpose of the spiral fold is to retard the movement of the intestinal contents and to increase the area of the secretory and absorbing surface. As a structural modification possessing this character we saw the fold in the Cyclostomata, Selachians and Dipnœans (Figs. 310, 466, 467 and 468) and in certain Ophidians (*Python* and *Anaconda*,Figs. 331 and 469). Among Mammals it is found in certain Rodentia in two forms:

(*a*) In some of the Muridæ, as *Arvicola* (Fig. 394), the mucous membrane of the large globular cæcal pouch is smooth, but the proximal segment of the colon, immediately beyond the ileo-colic junction, develops the spiral fold (Fig. 465, *IV*, 2).

(*b*) In other forms, as in the hares (Fig. 465, *IV*, 3), the greater part of the cæcum carries a typical spiral fold, continued up to the root of the terminal appendage (Fig. 388), in which segment the mucous membrane is devoid of folds, but studded thickly with lymphoid follicles. Beyond the cæcum proper the spiral fold is continued in the opposite direction into the proximal segment of the colon, which is large and capacious and evidently shares both the physiological and morphological characters of the cæcum proper, forming so to speak an accessory cæcal chamber. Beyond what we thus might term the cæcal division of the colon the large intestine becomes reduced in caliber, and the previously continuous spiral fold becomes broken up into separate semilunar haustral plicæ, corresponding to the superficial constrictions between the colic cells. In structure this distal segment of the rabbit colon closely resembles the human large intestine (Fig. 474).

One of the most marked examples of this secondary modification of the colon is presented by the intestinal canal of another Rodent, *Lagomys pusillus* (Fig. 391).

The cæcum of this animal is long, curved, provided with a well-developed spiral fold. The terminal segment of the pouch is reduced to an appendix, with smooth mucosa containing adenoid tissue, as in the rabbit. A second adenoid appendix, representing the globular saccus lymphaticus of the rabbit, is derived from the cæcum at the ileo-colic junction. The first segment of the colon beyond the ileo-colic junction is dilated and sacculated, the cæcal mucous fold being prolonged into it. This is succeeded by a narrow smooth-walled second segment. The third division of the colon is again dilated and sacculated, followed by a short fourth smooth-walled section. A fifth stretch is again provided with colic cells, beyond which the terminal segment continues of uniform caliber

122

and with smooth walls to the vent. The colon therefore presents three distinct sacculated portions whose structural modifications suggest that they function in the same sense as the cæcal pouch proper. In man and in other Primates the crescentic colic plicæ are disposed in a more or less evident spiral manner around the axis of the intestine, and it is not difficult to recognize in them the modified remnants of the typical spiral valve of lower forms. On the other hand, in conformity with the general reduction of the cæcal apparatus, the mucous membrane of the large intestine in Carnivora is smooth and devoid of any trace of the spiral fold (Fig. 475).

2. The second structural modification of the large intestine, associated in functional significance with the cæcal apparatus, depends upon the increase in the length of the proximal segment of the colon beyond the ileo-colic junction and the twisting or coiling of this segment in a more or less complicated definite manner, usually in the form of a spiral, the individual turns of the coil being held in place by the peritoneal connections. The proximal colon thus modified is admirably adapted to retard the movement of contents not yet completely digested and to increase the absorbing surface of the intestine, and hence is functionally allied to the cæcal apparatus.

This colic modification is found in its highest degree of development in the ruminant Ungulates, whose cæcal pouch proper is also enormously developed. In these animals the colon immediately beyond the ileo-cæcal junction is arranged in the form of a double spiral, the afferent (cæcal) and efferent (colic) tubes alternating, and continuous with each other in the center of the coil (Fig. 465, *IV*, 5). Examples of this type of spiral colon are shown in Fig. 373 (*Bos indicus*), Fig. 374 (*Cervus sika*), Fig. 375 (*Ovis aries*), Fig. 376 (*Oryx leucoryx*). Ontogenetically the complicated spiral colon of the ruminants starts as a simple loop of the proximal colon, which, with the further rapid growth of this segment of the intestine, is bent to produce the turns of the coil as shown in the schematic Figs. 480-482. Phylogenetically the same gradual development can be traced in the vertebrate series. Perhaps the earliest tendency to structurally modify the intestine in the direction named is found in the manner in which the intestinal coils are bound together by the subperitoneal arachnoid in many Ophidians (Fig. 331). Further in the Manidæ among the Edentates there is no cæcal pouch, but the intestine at the ileo-colic junction is twisted into a figure 8 and held in this position by the peritoneal connections (Figs. 362 and 465, *IV*, 4). In certain Marsupials with well-developed cæcal pouches, such as *Phascolarctos* and the Vulpine Phalangers (Figs. 351 and 352), the colon immediately beyond the ileo-colic entrance is sacculated and bent in the form of a short loop. In the tapir (Fig. 377), the proximal segment of the colon forms a simple loop, whose afferent and efferent limbs are closely bound together. The arrangement of the large intestine in this animal illustrates the early embryonal stage in the development of the complete ruminant spiral coil (cf. Fig. 480).

FIGS. 480-482.—Schematic representation of three stages in the development of the ungulate spiral colon.

The condition encountered in some Rodents presents a more advanced stage. Thus the large intestine in the agouti (*Dasyprocta agouti*), shows the development of the spiral coil advanced as far as the second turn of the original loop (Figs. 389 and 390). It is readily seen that continued growth of this segment of the intestine leads to the formation of the complete colic spiral as found in the typical Ungulates.

The same arrangement of the large intestine obtains in certain Lemurs among the Primates. Thus the proximal colon of the Slow Lemur (*Nycticebus tardigradus*) is seen in Figs. 421 and 422 to present a typical spiral coil, and similar conditions are encountered in other members of the suborder.

V. Cæcal Apparatus and Colon in Hyrax.

FIGS. 483-485.—Schematic figures illustrating possible line of derivation of aberrant mammalian type of alimentary canal encountered in *Hyrax*.

We have left for our final consideration the aberrant and unique mammalian type found in *Hyrax* (Fig. 378). In this remarkable little animal the large intestine develops a typical mammalian sacculated cæcum at the ileo-colic junction, and in addition is provided further on with two symmetrical pointed lateral colic cæca of large size. It is quite true that this arrangement is unique among Mammalia, confined entirely to the members of the suborder formed by the single family of *Hyrax*, and that no strictly analogous disposition of the alimentary canal is encountered in the entire vertebrate series. Yet these aberrant structures are possibly capable of explanation, in regard to the method of their development, by reference to the cæcal apparatus of certain phytophagous saurians, as *Iguana* and*Cyclura*. In these forms (Fig. 326-330) the small intestine enters the colon somewhat asymmetrically, the opening being guarded by a well developed annular valve.

The proximal segment of the large intestine forms an extensive sacculated pouch. If this is opened (Figs. 328-330) it is seen that the small intestine leads into a compartment which is separated from the remainder of the pouch by a valvular diaphragm with central circular opening. Beyond this primary compartment the colic pouch is incompletely subdivided by a series of gradually diminishing crescentic folds, corresponding to the external constrictions between the sacculations. The entire pouch gradually diminishes in caliber until it passes with a sharp angular bend into the terminal portion of the endgut. This terminal segment is differentiated from the elongated colic pouch by the greater thickness of its muscular walls and by a slight annular projecting fold in the interior. In considering the intestinal tract of *Hyrax* it is conceivable that the unique condition presented by this animal may be derived from some type conforming in general structure to the reptilian arrangement of the parts just detailed, as indicated in the schematic Figs. 483-485. The proximal typical cæcal pouch of *Hyrax* would then correspond to the similar colic pouch of *Iguana*. To explain the supplementary colic cæca it is necessary to suppose that the transition of the colic pouch into the terminal hindgut had become well differentiated, and that on each side of this junction the colic tube had extended backwards, resulting in the production of the supplementary bilateral cæcal pouches of *Hyrax*.

PART IV.
MORPHOLOGY OF THE HUMAN CÆCUM AND VERMIFORM APPENDIX.

Not only is the anatomy of this portion of the alimentary tract of great interest in relation to the evolution of the human structure, but in addition the pathological and surgical importance of the region warrants a very careful study of the cæcum and appendix. This is more especially the case since a number of variations in the arrangement of the structures are encountered. These departures from what we consider the normal human type have an important bearing on the development and progress of the pathological conditions prone to involve the appendix. We may consider the subject under the following subdivisions:

I. DEVELOPMENT OF THE CÆCUM AND APPENDIX.

Much light is thrown on the adult anatomy of the parts and on the origin of the variations observed by the study of their embryonic history. In considering the factors which determine the variations in the position, size, and shape of the appendix it must be remembered that the rudimentary character of this structure is responsible for many of the aberrant conditions encountered.

As a part of the general cæcal pouch which persists in an early developmental stage and which we can regard as destined for further reduction and ultimate elimination in the course of evolution, the appendix shares with other vestigial structures a wide range of variation. Consequently the study of the development of this portion of the alimentary tract enables us to gain a clearer view of the primary arrangement of the structures and to trace the causes which are active in determining the adult conditions most frequently encountered.

FIG. 486.—Alimentary canal and appendages of human embryo of 12.5 mm. × 12. (Kollmann, after His.)

FIG. 487.—*A*, schematic representation of alimentary canal, with umbilical loop and mesenteric attachments in human embryo of about six weeks. *B* and *C*, stages in the intestinal rotation.

At the time when the umbilical loop of the intestine has formed and has begun to protrude into the cavity of the umbilical cord (fifth to sixth week), the first indication of the future cæcum appears as a circumscribed thickening of the returning or ascending limb of the intestinal loop a short distance from the apex (Figs. 486-488). This rudiment indicates the derivation of the future definite intestinal segments from the elements of the loop. The descending limb, apex (site of embryonic vitelline duct, Meckel's diverticulum of adult) and a short succeeding portion of the ascending limb furnish the ileum and jejunum. The rest of the ascending limb develops into cæcum and appendix, ascending and transverse colon. The increase in the length of the intestine is not uniform. The formation of convolutions begins in the seventh week in the apex and subsequently in the descending limb. By the eighth week a considerable number of jejuno-ileal coils have resulted from the growth in length of these parts of the original umbilical loop, while the growth of the segment which furnishes the colon is at this time still inconsiderable (Fig. 489). In the meanwhile the thickening of the tube which forms the first rudiment of the cæcum has developed into a small sac-like enlargement of the gut, budding from the left and dorsal aspect of the ascending limb, crescentic in shape, turning its concavity toward the parent tube. In the majority of instances examined the small outgrowth is packed closely between the incipient ileal convolutions, lying under cover of the more prominent bulging coils of the umbilical protrusion, between them and a single coil of larger arc situated dorsally and belonging to the jejunal or proximal portion of the small intestine (Fig. 490). Fig. 497, taken from an embryo of 11 mm. cervico-coccygeal length, represents this stage in the development of the umbilical loop. The arrangement of the cæcum which we can assume as the typical condition at this stage and which determines in part the subsequent final arrangement of the structures, is illustrated by this relation of the cæcal bud to the surrounding incipient convolutions of the small intestine, with the larger part of these coils situated ventrad of the cæcum and only a single coil of larger curve placed dorsally; the cæcal pouch, derived from the ascending limb of the umbilical loop, is situated between these two divisions, turning its concave border to the right and embracing the parent tube. At the time when the human cæcum first appears as a distinct structure it forms a small conical pouch with blunt extremity whose shape is well illustrated by the cæcum of some of the new-world monkeys, as *Mycetes fuscus*, the brown howler monkey (Figs. 449 and 450). The outgrowth develops rapidly in length and very soon assumes a distinct crescentic shape, gradually tapering toward the extremity, a type which is found reproduced in the cæcum of *Ateles ater*, the black-handed spider monkey (Fig. 443). There is as yet no constriction or demarcation separating the distal segment (future appendix) from the proximal part (cæcum proper) but the entire pouch gradually narrows funnel-like to its termination.

FIGS. 488-492.—Series of schematic figures illustrating stages in the rotation of the intestinal canal.

FIGS. 493-496.—Series of schematic figures illustrating stages in the rotation of the intestinal canal.

II. CHANGES IN THE POSITION OF THE CÆCUM AND APPENDIX DURING NORMAL DEVELOPMENT, DEPENDING UPON THE ROTATION OF THE INTESTINE AND THE SUBSEQUENT DESCENT OF THE CÆCUM.

The primary cause leading to the rotation of the intestinal canal and inaugurating the successive stages which produce the adult disposition of the tube is to be found in the rapid increase in length of the small intestine. Numerous convolutions of this tube succeed to the few primary coils noted in the first stages. This condition is illustrated in Fig. 498, taken from an embryo of 4.4 cm. cervico-coccygeal measure, and the arrangement of the intestine is indicated in schema, Fig. 491. The cæcum is found nearly in the median line imbedded among the surrounding coils of the small intestine, which by their rapid increase have pushed the pouch cephalad nearly into contact with the caudal surface of the liver.

FIG. 497.—Human embryo of 11 mm. cervico-coccygeal measure. Enlarged view of ventral and left aspect of intestinal canal.

FIG. 498.—Human embryo of 4.4 cm. cervico-coccygeal measure. Intestinal canal; Liver removed. (Columbia University, Study Collection.)

Three main divisions of the convolutions of the small intestine can be made out, slightly separated from each other in the figure to exhibit the cæcum between them. The proximal (jejunal) set of these convolutions occupy the upper and left part of the abdominal cavity. They are the product of the single larger coil which in the earlier stage (Fig. 497, schemaFig. 490) appeared dorsad of the cæcal diverticulum. The distal (ileal) division of small intestinal convolutions has become greatly augmented and lies to the right of the cæcum. The concavity of the pouch is still, as in the earlier stages, directed to the right and the entrance of ileum into colon takes place from right to left. The caudal part of the abdominal cavity is occupied by an intermediate set of transition convolutions which join the proximal and distal divisions. In the two stages just described (Figs. 497 and 498, Schema Figs. 490and 491), the initial step in the intestinal rotation has been taken, *i. e.*, the beginning of the colon has been displaced cephalad from its original position in the caudal and left part of the abdominal cavity by the pressure of the rapidly growing coils of the small intestine and now lies transversely ventrad of the duodenum, having crossed the duodeno-colic neck or isthmus of the primitive umbilical loop (cf. Fig. 487, *C*).

At first the distal coils of the small intestine occupy a position *behind* as well as to the right of the cæcum, forming a dorsal retro-cæcal division connected by intermediate convolutions with the ventral division occupying the lower and left portion of the abdominal cavity. The apex of the cæcum is frequently imbedded among these terminal coils of the ileum. With the continued growth of the small intestines a further displacement of the cæcum cephalad and to the right takes place, while at the same time the terminal ileal coils pass downwards and to the left, from a retro-cæcal into a subcæcal position, thus permitting a direct apposition of the cæcum to the dorsal parietal (prerenal) peritoneum. The last steps in this process of withdrawal of the original voluminous dorsal (retro-cæcal) division of ileal convolutions are well seen in the preparation shown in Fig. 499, taken from an embryo of 6.7 cm. vertex-coccygeal measure, and corresponding to the schematic stages represented in Figs. 490 and491. The cæcum in this preparation has not yet completed its rotation and still turns its concavity upwards and to the right, with the apex imbedded among the terminal convolutions of the ileum.

FIG. 499.—Human embryo of 6.7 cm. vertex-coccygeal measure. Liver removed. (Columbia University, Study Collection.)

FIG. 500.—Human embryo of 4.9 cm. vertex-coccygeal measure. Ventral view of abdominal cavity, with liver partially removed. (Columbia University, Study Collection.)

FIG. 501.—The same embryo represented in Fig. 500. The colic coil further depressed and turned to the left; seen from the right side.

The ileo-cæcal junction takes place from right to left in a downward direction. Nearly the entire mass of the small intestine is situated below and to the left of cæcum and colon, but a terminal ileal coil still occupies, although evidently in the process of withdrawal, the retro-cæcal position, separating the cæcum from direct contact with the dorsal parietal peritoneum. The withdrawal of this terminal coil of the small intestine is accompanied, or immediately followed, by a further turn of the colon cephalad and to the right, which brings it into contact with the caudal surface of the liver and completes the rotation, producing a change in the relative positions of the terminal ileal coils and the cæcum. In the stages illustrated in Figs. 498 and 499 and shown schematically in Figs. 490 and491, the terminal coils of the ileum pass from right to left behind the cæcum to enter the colon, and the concavity of the cæcal pouch is directed upwards and to the right. After the final rotation has occurred (schema,Fig. 492) the ileum enters the large intestine from the left and from below, and the concave border of the cæcum is directed caudad and to the left. This change in relative position has been accomplished by a revolution of the colon and cæcum through an arc of 180° around its own long axis carrying the cæcum above and behind the small intestine and bringing it into contact with the dorsal prerenal parietal peritoneum. At the same time the terminal coils of the ileum turn downwards and to the left. If this final step in the rotation of the large intestine fails to occur, with otherwise normal development of the parts, the ileum will persist in entering the large intestine from right to left after the cæcum has obtained its final lodgment in the right iliac fossa. We have had occasion to refer previously to the significance of these instances of partially arrested development (cf.p. 61, Figs. 123, 127 and 128).

In Figs. 500 and 501, taken from an embryo of 4.9 cm. vertex-coccygeal measure, the final rotation of the cæcum from the position occupied in Fig. 498 has occurred and the concavity of the pouch is directed caudad and towards the left. At the same time the escape of the terminal ileal coils from behind the cæcum and beginning of the colon has not yet taken place and hence the colon is still kept by these coils from direct opposition to the dorsal prerenal parietal peritoneum. The condition presented by this preparation can be schematically indicated by Figs. 492 and 493. The rotation has carried the beginning of the colon (Fig. 500), with the cæcal bud and appendix curved on itself and turning its concavity to the left, into the subhepatic position. The greater part of the small intestinal coils lie now below and to the left of the cæcum, but the terminal ileal convolutions (Fig. 500) still occupy a retro-cæcal position, separating the pouch and the colon from the dorsal parietal peritoneum. In Fig. 501 the right lateral view of the same embryo is shown with the cæcum and colon depressed and turned to the left. The termination of the ileum reaches the ileocolic junction by passing behind the cæcum, and the immediately adjacent ileal coils are still retro-cæcal, intervening between the pouch and the dorsal parietal peritoneum.

In the next succeeding stage (schema, Fig. 494) these coils of the ileum turn downward and to the left so as to lie below and mesad to the cæcum and colon, thus permitting the direct apposition of the large intestine to the parietal prerenal peritoneum. The terminal ileum now passes from below and to the left upwards and to the right to its junction with the colon. This freeing of the dorsal surface of cæcum and colon from contact with the coils of the small intestines, and the consequent direct apposition of the same to the dorsal parietal peritoneum influences to a great extent the subsequent arrangement of the parts, because it affords the conditions necessary to the fixation of the colon and mesocolon by adhesion to the parietal peritoneum (cf. p. 81).

Fig. 499, taken from an embryo of 6.7 cm. vertex-coccygeal measure, illustrates this stage, which is encountered in the majority of instances and during which the retro-cæcal coils of the terminal ileum are withdrawn (schema, Fig. 493). The convolutions of the small intestine have greatly increased in size and number. The retro-cæcal ileal coils, compared with Fig. 500, have shifted their position caudad and to the left, so as to lie below and ventrad of the beginning of the colon. Only a single coil remains behind the cæcum and appendix, intervening between these structures and the ventral surface of the right kidney, and this coil is in the process of withdrawal from the dorsal position as indicated by the superficial and short course of the coil which connects it with the remaining ventral convolutions. As soon as the withdrawal of this single remaining dorsal coil is completed the entire mass of the small intestines will occupy a position ventrad, caudad and to the left of the cæcum and colon (Fig. 494), which will then rest directly against the dorsal parietal peritoneum investing the ventral surface of the right kidney.

FIG. 502.—Human embryo, 6.6 cm. vertex-coccygeal measure. Liver removed. (Columbia University, Study Collection.)

This stage is illustrated in Fig. 502, taken from an embryo of 6.6 cm. vertex-coccygeal measure. The cæcum and appendix here occupy the subhepatic position, well to the right of the median line and in the background of the abdominal cavity. The terminal retro-cæcal ileal coils of the embryo shown in Figs. 500 and 501 have descended caudad and to the left, thus freeing the dorsal surface of cæcum and colon and permitting direct contact with the prerenal parietal peritoneum.

In the succeeding stages the cæcum gradually descends along the background of the right lumbar region from the subhepatic position to the right iliac fossa, producing by this descent the ascending colon as a distinct segment of the large intestine.

It will be observed that in the stage shown in Fig. 502 (schema, Fig. 494) the large intestine passes from the cæcum to the splenic flexure transversely from right to left across the upper part of the abdominal cavity, caudad and ventrad of the stomach and cephalad of the coils of the small intestine.

In the following stages the disproportionately large size of the embryonic liver compels the colon, as the cæcum descends, to assume an oblique position. When the cæcal descent is completed the colon traverses the abdominal cavity in contact with the caudal surface of the liver passing from the right iliac fossa obliquely cephalad and to the left to the splenic flexure where it becomes continuous with the descending colon, which segment has early assumed its definite position in the background of the abdominal cavity on the left side (Fig. 495). This oblique position of the colon is seen in Figs. 503 and 504. During this stage the increase in the length of the colon may lead to the arrangement seen in Fig. 505, where the future transverse segment of the large intestine is bent caudad in form of an arch whose summit extends nearly to the pelvis. This condition at times persists in the adult, in cases of unusually long large intestine, and recalls the normal arrangement found in many of the cynomorphous monkeys in whom the transverse colon forms an extensive V-or U-shaped loop, with the apex directed caudad toward the pubic symphysis (Fig. 506). In other instances in the human fœtus this part of the large intestine is thrown into a number of shorter irregular coils (Fig. 507).

FIG. 503.—Human embryo, 7.6 cm. vertex-coccygeal measure. Liver and small intestine from the duodeno-jejunal to the junction removed. (Columbia University, Study Collection.)

FIG. 504.—Human fœtus, 10.6 cm. vertex-coccygeal measure. Liver and greater part of small intestine removed. (Columbia University, Study Collection.)

FIG. 505.—Human fœtus, 20.4 cm. vertex-coccygeal measure. (Columbia University, Study Collection.)

FIG. 507.—Abdominal viscera of human fœtus at term, hardened *in situ*; hepatic flexure formed, and ascending and transverse colon differentiated. (Columbia University Museum, No. 1816.)

FIG. 506.—Abdominal viscera of *Macacus rhesus*, rhesus monkey, hardened *in situ*. (Columbia University Museum, No 1817.)

FIG. 508.—Human fœtus of 10.7 cm. vertex-coccygeal measure. Liver and small intestine from the duodeno-jejunal to the ileo-colic junction removed. The colon already presents an ascending, transverse and descending segment. The appendix is retro-cæcal, curved, with the tip turned down, under cover of the ileo-colic junction and mesentery. (Columbia University, Study Collection.)

Normally, however, in the process of further development and with the relative decrease in the size of the liver, the hepatic flexure (Fig. 505) becomes defined and passes cephalad and to the right, taking up the slack of the bent segment and establishing the typical ascending and transverse colon as seen in Fig. 508 (schema, Fig. 496).

III. VARIATIONS OF ADULT CÆCUM AND APPENDIX.

The study of the variations of the adult cæcum and appendix involves the consideration of the following points:

(*a*) Shape of cæcum and origin of appendix. (*Type of adult cæcum.*)

(*b*) Position, direction and peritoneal relations of the appendix.

(*c*) Arrangement of the vascular and serous ileo-cæcal folds.

The peculiarities encountered in any individual case usually depend upon the combination of all three of these factors, which together influence and determine the

128

arrangement of the structures in the adult. Hence the examination of each case should be made with reference to these three points, which we will now consider in detail.

A. SHAPE OF CÆCUM AND ORIGIN OF APPENDIX. TYPES AND VARIATIONS OF ADULT CÆCUM AND APPENDIX.

The various forms of the adult cæcum are all derived by modifications from the fœtal type of the pouch.

In the embryo the cæcum is funnel-shaped, narrowing gradually and symmetrically in caliber to the root of the appendix, at which point the three colic tænia or longitudinal muscular bands of the large intestine meet. The appendix arises from the apex of the funnel, the lateral walls of which are equally and symmetrically developed. The entire pouch is of a crescentic shape, the concavity of the curve turned to the left and directed toward the caudal margin of the terminal ileum. Two subdivisions of the fœtal type are found:

FIG. 509.—Schematic table of types of human cæca.

FIG. 510.—Human fœtus at term. Cæcum and ileo-colic junction; ventral view. (Columbia University, Study Collection.)

1. Appendix.
2. Reduced intermediate non-vascular fold.
3. Ventral vascular fold.

I. The crescentic curve of the cæcum is only slightly marked; the appendix arises from the most pendent part of the pouch and hangs downward (schema, Fig. 509, I, a).

This form, which is encountered only occasionally in the fœtus and infant, is illustrated by the preparation shown in Fig. 510, taken from a fœtus at term.

II. In the majority of cases the inherent crescentic shape of the cæcal pouch is pronounced and carries the termination of the funnel with the root of the appendix cephalad and to the left toward the caudal margin of the ileo-colic junction (schema, Fig. 509, II, a).

At birth this typical arrangement of the cæcum frequently places the pouch in a nearly transverse position, with the apex and the root of the appendix turned to the left, in contact with, or under cover of the terminal piece of the ileum at its junction with the large intestine.

Figs. 511 and 512 represent the parts in the ventral view in the fœtus at term.

FIG. 511.—Human fœtus at term. Cæcum and ileo-colic junction; ventral view. (Columbia University, Study Collection.)

1. Appendix, coiled spirally behind terminal ileum.
2. Non-vascular intermediate fold.

FIG. 512.—Human fœtus at term (negro). Cæcum and ileo-colic junction; ventral view. (Columbia University Museum, No. 692.)

FIG. 513.—Human fœtus at term. Cæcum and ileo-colic junction; dorsal view. (Columbia University, Study Collection.)

FIG. 514.—Human fœtus at term. Cæcum and ileo-colic junction; dorsal view. (Columbia University Museum, No. 1715.)

Figs. 513 and 514, also taken from the fœtus at term, show the cæcum from the dorsal aspect and illustrate well the sharp character of the curve which carries the apex of the pouch up and to the left.

All the variations observed in the adult cæcum are derived from these two fœtal types by a subsequent and usually asymmetrical enlargement and dilatation of the pouch.

We can consider the derivatives of each form separately.

I. Adult Cæca Derived From Type I. (schema, Fig. 509, I^a, Fig. 510).

1. Further development leads to an enlargement of the cæcal pouch and a sharper demarcation between the same and the appendix. The resulting cæcum is symmetrical, with equally developed lateral sacculi, between which the termination of the longitudinal muscular bands and the root of the appendix is situated (schema, Fig. 509, I^b).

FIG. 515.—Human fœtus at term. Cæcum and ileo-colic junction; ventral view. (Columbia University Museum, No. 1510.)

FIG. 516.—Human fœtus at term. Cæcum and ileo-colic junction; ventral view. (Columbia University Museum, No. 1548.)

In Figs. 515 and 516 two infantile cæca are shown which illustrate this form. The narrow and pointed apex of the fœtal conical cæcum is replaced by the capacious pouch which is differentiated sharply from the appendix. Among the anthropoid apes the same type is seen in the cæcum of the gibbon (Figs. 455 and 456), and of the young chimpanzee shown in Fig. 460.

2. An increased development of the cæcal pouch in the adult leads to the protrusion caudad of two symmetrical sacculations on each side of the root of the appendix which appears between them. The original apex of the cæcal pouch is still marked by the implantation of the appendix and by the termination of the longitudinal muscular bands, but the lowest level of the pouch is found on each side of this point at the fundus of the secondary lateral sacculi (schema, Fig. 509, I). Treves, to whom belongs the credit of first accurately describing and classifying the forms of the adult cæcum based on the development, found this type in three of a series of 100 cases examined.

FIG. 517.—Adult human cæcum and ileo-colic junction. (Columbia University, Study Collection.)

FIG. 518.—Adult human cæcum and ileo-colic junction. (Columbia University Museum, No. 234.)

Figs. 517 and 518 illustrate this form of the pouch, which, in our experience, is frequently associated with the retro-cæcal erect position of the appendix (cf. infra, p. 251). Fig. 472 shows this type in the adult with pendent appendix.

II. Adult Cæca Derived from Type II. (schema, Figs. 509 and 511).—From this more commonly observed type of fœtal cæcum the following adult forms are developed:

1. The general shape and trend of the fœtal cæcum is preserved. The pouch turns sharply to the left, carrying the apex with the root of the appendix upward toward the ileum, the appendix itself being frequently placed under cover of the terminal coil of the small intestine (schema, Fig. 509, II^{b}).

FIG. 519.—Human adult (Smith's Sound Eskimo). Ileo-colic junction and cæcum. (Columbia University Museum, No. 59/1483.)

FIG. 520.—Human adult. Ileo-colic junction and cæcum. (Columbia University, Study Collection.)

FIG. 521.—Human adult. Ileo-colic junction and cæcum. (Columbia University, Study Collection.)

FIG. 522.—Human adult (Smith's Sound Eskimo). Ileo-colic junction and cæcum. (Columbia University Museum, No. 56/1571.)

The apex of the cæcal pouch is either conical, narrowing gradually toward the root of the appendix (Figs. 520 and 521), or blunt and more sharply defined against the appendix (Fig. 522). Mr. Treves encountered this "persistent fœtal type" in two per cent. of his series.

FIG. 523.—Human adult. Ileo-colic junction and cæcum; dorsal view; dried preparation. (Columbia University Museum, No. 200.)

FIG. 524.—Human fœtus at term. Ileo-colic junction and cæcum; ventral view. (Columbia University Museum, No. 1717.)

FIG. 525.—Same preparation as Fig. 524; dorsal view.

The cæcum is frequently sharply bent on itself in making the turn upward and to the left, resulting in a deep indentation of the concave border and producing a corresponding projecting fold in the interior of the pouch (Fig. 523). The ventral longitudinal muscular band follows the crescentic sweep of the cæcum to the root of the appendix.

Figs. 524a and 525b, representing the cæcum of a fœtus at term in the ventral and dorsal view respectively, show very clearly the arrangement of the fœtal pouch from which the adult type with sharp angular bend is derived. This type of adult cæcum is found in certain of the anthropoid apes.

In the orang (Figs. 458 and 459) the cæcum turns sharply upward and to the left, gradually narrowing in caliber to the root of the appendix which is coiled behind the termination of the ileum.

130

The same type is seen in Figs. 462 and 463, taken from a preparation of the adult chimpanzee. Fig. 463 shows especially well the sharp bend between the cæcum and colon by means of which the apex of the pouch is carried cephalad behind the ileo-colic junction.

Fig. 431, taken from another specimen of the same animal, shows the characteristic crescentic curve of the cæcum and the corresponding course of the longitudinal muscular band. The apex of the pouch in this preparation is more rounded and blunt.

The same blunt termination of the cæcum of this type, with a corresponding sharper demarcation of the appendix, is seen in the gorilla (Fig. 457) recalling the conditions found in certain instances in the human subject (Fig. 522).

2. In by far the larger proportion of cases (ninety per cent. in Treves' series) the adult cæcum obtains its characteristic form by an unequal development of the walls of the intestine. The right segment between the ventral and dorso-lateral muscular bands, forming a sacculation which projects caudad and constitutes the secondary caput coli, while the segment between the lower border of the ileum and the original apex, marked by the origin of the appendix, remains stationary or is further reduced. This unequal development produces a relative displacement of the root of the appendix upward and to the left toward the ileo-colic junction.

In some cases the primitive crescentic curve of the cæcum, as indicated by the direction of the ventral longitudinal muscular band, is still perceptible.

The right wall of the fœtal cæcum, forming the most pendent portion of the pouch, dilates uniformly and thus constitutes the adult caput coli. The left wall appears as a small sacculation separating the root of the appendix from the ileo-colic junction (schema, Fig. 509, *II, c*). This type of the adult cæcum is illustrated by the preparations shown in Figs. 526-528. In other cases part of the right wall of the cæcum between the ventral and dorso-lateral colic tænia, dilates abruptly forming a very prominent rounded sacculation which carries the lowest part of the pouch caudad in a sharper curve than in the preceding form as indicated by its deviation from the direction of the longitudinal muscular band (schema, Fig. 509, *II, d*).

FIG. 526.—Human adult (Smith's Sound Eskimo). Ileo-colic junction and cæcum; dorsal view. (Columbia University Museum, No. 61/1461.)

FIG. 527.—Human adult. Ileo-colic junction and cæcum; ventral view. (Columbia University, Study Collection.)

FIG. 528.—Human adult. Ileo-colic junction and cæcum; ventral view. (Columbia University, Study Collection.)

Figs. 529-531 afford examples of this type, while Fig. 532, taken from an infantile preparation, shows that the same may begin to develop at a very early age.

FIG. 530.—Human adult. Ileo-colic junction and cæcum; dorsal view. (Columbia University Museum, No. 115.)

FIG. 529.—Human juvenile. Ileo-colic junction and cæcum; dorsal view. (Columbia University, Study Collection.)

FIG. 531.—Human adult. Ileo-colic junction and cæcum; dorsal view. (Columbia University, Study Collection.)

FIG. 532.—Human infant, Ileo-colic junction and cæcum, with secondary terminal sacculation. Human infant, Ileo-colic junction and cæcum, with secondary terminal sacculation. (Columbia University Museum, No. 1632.)

3. Finally, in about four per cent. to five per cent., adult cæca, the reduction of the wall to the left of the root of the appendix, between this point and the ileo-colic junction, is complete. The entire cæcal pouch is formed by the dilated right wall between the ventral and dorsolateral muscular bands. The ventral band terminates at the lower border of the ileo-colic junction, from which the appendix appears to arise, indicating the original apex of the fœtal cæcum (schema, Fig. 509, *IIᵗ*).

This type is illustrated in the specimens shown in Figs. 533 and 534.

FIG. 534.—Human adult. Ileo-colic junction and cæcum; ventral view; dried preparation. (Columbia University Museum,

FIG. 533.—Human adult. Ileo-colic

junction and cæcum; dorsal view; dried   No. 14.)
preparation. (Columbia University Museum,
No. 124.)

III. Adult Cæca in Cases of Absence of the Appendix.—A few instances of congenital absence of the appendix have been observed.

FIG. 535.—Human adult. Ileo-colic junction and cæcum; absence of appendix. (Columbia University Museum, No. 1077.)

FIG. 536.—Human adult. Ileo-colic junction and cæcum, hardened *in situ*; absence of appendix. (Columbia University Museum, No. 715.)

A. v. Haller[9] describes the condition in the following words: "Defuisse visa est in homine appendicula, ut tuberculum minimum superesset."

Fr. Arnold,[10] without describing any individual case, states that "very rarely the appendix is entirely wanting."

E. Zuckerkandl,[11] reports having observed one case of absence of the appendix.

J. D. Bryant,[12] reports a case in which he operated for appendicitis but found "absolutely no appendix." "The point of tenderness was found to be a glandular growth located posterior to the usual site of the appendix."

Two instances of this variation are shown in Figs. 535 and 536, taken from preparations in the Morphological Museum of Columbia University. In both careful examination of the external as well as of the mucous surface of the cæcum demonstrated the entire absence of the appendix, and the subjects from which they were obtained presented no scars or other evidences of operative removal or of pathological processes. They are both, therefore, authentic instances of complete congenital absence of the appendix, not of so-called retro-peritoneal or hidden appendix.[13]

The two examples differ from each other in some details. In the first case (Fig. 535, schema, Fig. 509, *III*[a]) the cæcum is rounded and globular. The ventral longitudinal muscular band is vertical and continued to the lowest point of the pouch, which greatly resembles the cæcum of a typical cynomorphous monkey.

In the second case (Fig. 536, schema, Fig. 509, *III*[b]) the cæcum turns upwards and to the left, terminating in a sharp point, to which several lobes of epiploic fat are attached.

We must assume that in these cases the embryonic portion of the cæcal bud was developed just sufficiently to yield the required adult pouch with nothing to spare, so to speak, which could remain rudimentary in the form of an appendix.

Instances of exceedingly rudimentary and reduced appendix are also encountered.

In the case illustrated in Fig. 537 the appendix formed a small conical elevation without distinct lumen, measuring only 0.5 cm. in length.

FIG. 537.—Human adult. Ileo-colic junction and cæcum, with rudimentary appendix. (Columbia University Museum, No. 1655.)

B. Position and Peritoneal Relations of the Appendix.—Statistical records of the position of the appendix indicate a wide range of variation. In general the results obtained by different observers show that certain positions of the appendix are encountered in a sufficiently large percentage of the cases to enable us to adopt a classification, but that a very extensive series of records are required in order to determine even approximately the preponderant relations of the appendix. The following are the most frequently observed positions:

1. The appendix is directed upward, inward and to the left, the terminal portion being frequently coiled under cover of the ileum and mesentery. This position of the appendix is largely due to the normal crescentic curve of the cæcum, which carries the apex of the pouch and the root of the appendix upward and to the left. Its production is, moreover, favored by the tendency of the adult cæcum to develop by dilatation of the ventral and right wall at the expense of the left side of the pouch, thus relatively shortening the interval between the origin of the appendix and the ileo-colic junction.

Examples of this commonly encountered position of the appendix are given in Figs. 512, 513, 514, 520, 521, 523 and 526.

FIG. 538.—Human juvenile. Cæcum *in situ* lifted up to show vertical course of appendix, situated behind cæcum and ascending colon. The large intestine has a free peritoneal dorsal surface, and the appendix is held in position by adhesion to the large intestine. (Columbia University, Study Collection.)

2. The appendix is erected vertically behind the cæcum and ascending colon and closely attached to the dorsal wall of the large intestine. In some instances the cæcum and colon, with the adherent vertical appendix, possess a free serous dorsal surface, not adherent to the parietal peritoneum (Figs. 529, 538,539 and 540). In other cases the ascending colon is fixed and the greater part of the retro-colic appendix is buried in the connective tissue which attaches the large intestine to the abdominal parietes (Fig. 517). Even in these cases, however, the dorsal surface of the cæcum and the root of the appendix retain their free serous investment.

FIG. 539.—Human adult. Ileo-colic junction and cæcum; dorsal view. (Columbia University Museum, No. 1594.)

FIG. 540.—Human adult. Ileo-colic junction and cæcum; dorsal view. (Columbia University Museum, No. 1850.)

3. The proximal part of the appendix turns upward and to the left in continuation of the cæcal curve, but the distal portion is directed downward and inward, hanging over the brim of the pelvis (Figs. 505, 541 and 542).

FIG. 541.—Human infant. Ileo-colic junction and cæcum; ventral view. (Columbia University, Study Collection.)

FIG. 542.—Human infant. Ileo-colic junction and cæcum; dorsal view. The dorsal surface of cæcum as far as root of the appendix is adherent to the parietal peritoneum of the iliac fossa. (Columbia University Museum, No. 394.)

4. The appendix is directed downward, pendent from the lowest point of the conical cæcal pouch, and hangs free over the pelvic brim.

This type is encountered at times in fœtal and infantile subjects (Figs. 516 and 543).

FIG. 543.—Human fœtus at fifth month. Abdominal cavity and viscera; liver and greater part of small intestine removed. (Drawn from preparation in Columbia University Museum, No. 1814.)

FIG. 544.—Human fœtus at term. Abdominal cavity and viscera; greater part of small intestine removed. (Drawn from preparation in Columbia University Museum, No. 1813.)

FIG. 545.—Human fœtus at term. Ileo-colic junction and cæcum. (Columbia University Museum, No. 998.)

5. The position of the appendix is variant and abnormal, as *e. g.* placed to the right of cæcum and colon (Fig. 544) or turned up ventrad of the ileo-colic junction (Fig. 545).

These variations in the position of the appendix and the resulting peritoneal relations of the structure depend upon the following factors.

1. The influence of peritoneal adhesions established during the descent of the cæcum from the subhepatic position to the iliac fossa.

2. The inherent curve of the cæcal pouch.

3. The subsequent alterations in the caliber of the intestine and the unequal development of the pouch leading to the formation of the types of adult cæca above considered.

In determining the causes which lead to the establishment of any given position of the appendix all three of the factors above enumerated must be taken into account, although their influence is not exerted in every case to an equal degree.

We have seen that normally, after completed rotation of the intestine, the cæcum with the appendix and the beginning of the colon are lodged in the upper and right part of the abdomen, below the liver and in contact with the prerenal parietal peritoneum (schema,Figs. 493, 502). During the subsequent stages the cæcum descends into the right iliac fossa, thus producing the ascending colon. It is immaterial whether this change in position is regarded as an actual descent of the pouch over the ventral surface of the right kidney, which seems more probable, or as a growing away from the iliac region of the remainder of the abdominal wall, with a concomitant relative reduction in the size of the liver, producing a relatively lower position of the cæcum, or as a combination of these processes. In either case during this period the dorsal surface of the ascending colon and mesocolon normally becomes adherent to the dorsal parietal peritoneum, connective tissue developing between the opposed serous areas and leading to the usual fixation of the ascending colon and obliteration of the free ascending mesocolon. If this process of adhesion is inaugurated at an early stage, i. e., before the descent of the cæcum has been accomplished, it will act as a drag on the dorsal surface of the colic tube during the subsequent change in position, which carries the cæcum downward into the iliac fossa. This leads to a backward bend of the cæcum and appendix which parts will in the ventral view appear under cover of the protruding free ventral and lateral walls of the colon. Hence in many late embryos and fœtus at term the lowest point of the large intestine in the right iliac fossa is formed by the proximal part of the cæcum or by the adjacent segment of the colon, while the original termination of the pouch, with the root of the appendix, is turned backward and upward, and, as we have seen, by reason of the inherent shape of the pouch, also to the left, carrying the beginning of the appendix frequently behind the terminal ileum and the ileo-colic junction.

Two of the more common positions of the appendix, viz., backwards, upwards and inwards behind the ileo-colic junction, and directly backward, erected vertically behind cæcum and colon, can therefore in part be referred to the mechanical conditions obtaining normally during the descent of the cæcum. Of course the shape of the cæcal pouch and the later development of the adult type of cæcum will modify this influence in individual cases. We have seen that this early adhesion and the resulting effects on the position of cæcum and appendix depend on the direct apposition of the colic tube and mesocolon to the dorsal parietal peritoneum. Any condition which will prevent or delay this apposition will likewise perpetuate the original embryonal condition of the tube, completely invested by peritoneum and with a free mesocolon.

Such an element is found in the persistence of the dorsal set of ileal convolutions in the original retro-cæcal position beyond the usual period, as indicated in the schematic Fig. 492,IV, a. If the turn downward and to the left of these coils is for any reason delayed beyond the usual time the cæcal extremity of the colon will descend from the subhepatic to the iliac position without coming directly into contact with the dorsal parietal peritoneum, and therefore without the usual peritoneal adhesion and obliteration of the apposed serous surfaces. The cæcum under these conditions descends without making the backward bend, and the origin of the appendix is found at the lowest point of the pendent funnel-shaped pouch, causing it finally to hang downward or downward and inward over the pelvic brim. The resulting form of the cæcum and the position of the appendix is the one above described as type Ia, Ib and Ic (Fig. 509).

Fig. 510 from a fœtus at term, and Figs. 515 and 516 representing infantile cæca, illustrate this form of the pouch, while the parts are shown in situ in Fig. 543 taken from a preparation of a five-month fœtus.

FIG. 546.—Human embryo, 6.5 cm. cervico-coccygeal measure. Abdominal cavity, with liver removed, seen from the right side. (Columbia University, Study Collection.)

FIG. 547.—Human embryo, 5.9 cm. vertex-coccygeal measure. (Columbia University, Study Collection.)

FIG. 548.—Human fœtus at term. Ileo-colic junction and cæcum. Early colic and cæcal adhesion with retroverted appendix. (Columbia University Museum, Study Collection.)

Fig. 546 exhibits the condition obtaining during the development of this type in the more exceptional instances of delayed apposition of the colon to the parietal peritoneum and of increased development of the terminal ileal coils in the original retro-cæcal position. In this embryo, measuring 6.5 cm. in vertex-coccygeal length, the development has progressed sufficiently to establish a distinct transverse colon and to bring the cæcum and appendix into the subhepatic position. But in place of lying in contact with the dorsal parietal peritoneum, as in the embryo, shown in Fig. 502, over the ventral surface of the right kidney, the increased mass of the retro-cæcal ileal coils keeps the cæcum, already in the process of descent, in contact with the ventral abdominal wall. When the final rotation of the retro-cæcal small intestinal coils downward and to the left occurs, placing the ileo-colic junction (C) to the left of the large intestine (schema. Fig. 494), the ascending colon and cæcum are not yet fixed by adhesion to the dorsal parietal peritoneum, and the appendix will present downward and to the left, affording the necessary conditions for the establishment of the permanent pendent position of the tube or causing the same to be directed downward and inward over the brim of the pelvis.

In contrast with the preceding is the condition shown in Fig. 547, taken from an embryo of 5.9 cm. vertex-coccygeal measure. The transverse colon in this preparation has already begun to assume an oblique position, passing down and to the right from the splenic flexure. The cæcum and appendix are in contact with the dorsal prerenal parietal peritoneum. The escape of the dorsal set of ileal convolutions from the retro-cæcal position, by rotation downwards and to the left, is accomplished. The cæcum and appendix are placed in the position which they would have occupied in the embryo shown in Fig. 546 if the dorsal ileal coils had not prevented, in the latter preparation, the apposition of the colon to the dorsal parietal peritoneum.

In considering the effect of these variant conditions on the adult arrangement of the structures it is necessary to bear in mind the second of the above-mentioned factors, namely, the inherent shape of the cæcal pouch and appendix and the resulting direction of its axis.

As previously stated the normal type of the human embryonal cæcum is represented by the pouch of some of the new-world monkeys, as *Ateles* (Fig. 443) or of certain lemurs, of which *Nycticebus* (Fig. 420) furnishes an excellent example. The cæcum is distinctly crescentic, turning its concave margin, after completed intestinal rotation, upwards and to the left, toward the lower margin of the ileum. The distal diminished segment of the pouch in *Ateles* has already assumed the character of a cæcal appendage in *Nycticebus* and becomes by further reduction the typical appendix in man and the anthropoid apes, while the proximal portion develops into the capacious sacculated cæcum proper. Consequently the initial curve of the cæcum tends to carry the root of the appendix upward and to the left toward the ileo-colic junction. This curve of the pouch, combined with the mechanical effects produced by the adhesion of the colon during the cæcal descent, accounts for the frequency with which the cæcum in the later months of fœtal life and at birth is found curved backward, upward and to the left, placing the root of the appendix under cover of the terminal ileal convolutions (Fig. 548). We have seen that this disposition of the structures accounts for the preponderance of that type of adult cæcum which results from the further and unequal development and dilatation of the segment of the pouch situated to the right of the origin of the appendix.

Bearing in mind the three elements just considered, viz., the effect of adhesion during the cæcal descent, the inherent shape of the pouch and the unequal alterations in caliber in the development of the adult type, we can at once take up the resulting variations in the peritoneal relations of the adult cæcum and appendix which have an important influence on the progress of pathological processes in this region. It should be remembered that in the following schematic figures the colon, cæcum and appendix are represented in the profile view in a straight line, without indicating the characteristic turn of the crescentic cæcal pouch upwards and to the left.

Fig. 549 shows the arrangement in unimpeded cæcal descent without adhesion of colon and mesocolon to the parietal peritoneum. This disposition of the structures, if carried into adult life, would produce the permanently free ascending colon and mesocolon which we encountered exceptionally in the human subject (cf. p. 82) and normally in certain of the cynomorphous monkeys (p. 83). The ascending colon and mesocolon can, under these conditions, be turned mesad, lifting them away from the primary parietal peritoneum investing the ventral surface of the right kidney. Cæcum and appendix have, of course, a complete serous investment.

FIGS. 549-554.—Schematic series illustrating the variations in the arrangement of the cæcal and colic peritoneum.

FIG. 549. FIG. 550.

FIG. 551. FIG. 552.

FIG. 553. FIG. 554.

Normally, however, in the human subject, even if the obliteration of the apposed serous surfaces and the resulting fixation of the ascending colon has been delayed beyond the usual period, as above indicated, adhesion takes place subsequently, involving the dorsal surface of the ascending colon between the ileo-colic junction and the hepatic flexure (schema, Fig. 550). The dorsal surface of the cæcum usually retains its free serous surface in whole or in greater part. The appendix is pendent, entirely invested by peritoneum and hangs free in the abdominal cavity, directed toward the pelvic brim, illustrating the effect of delayed fixation of the colon on the position of the appendix.

Examples of this condition are not frequent, and are confined almost exclusively to fœtal and juvenile subjects. Illustrations are afforded by Figs. 515 and 516.

We have already noted (p. 246) the resulting fœtal type of pendent cæcum (Fig. 510).

More commonly colic adhesion before the cæcum obtains its final iliac position results in imparting a backward turn to the pouch, leading to the peritoneal disposition shown in schema, Fig. 551, in which the root of the appendix is involved in the area of obliteration, while the terminal segment remains free. An example of this condition is furnished by the embryo shown in Fig. 508 (10.7 cm. vertex-coccygeal measure). The colon is already segmented into an ascending, transverse and descending portion. The cæcum is retroverted and its apex with the appendix is placed under cover of the terminal ileum which enters the large intestine in the direction from below upward and to the right. In the side-figure the divided end of the ileum is displaced upward to show cæcum and appendix and their relation to the ileal mesentery.

The disposition of the structures illustrated by this example probably depends upon delayed adhesion of the colic embryonal tube to the dorsal parietal peritoneum. The cæcum and appendix appear to have descended freely until the final position in the right iliac fossa has been nearly attained, adhesion and fixation of the colon taking place just before the descent is completed, and thus producing the backward turn of the cæcal end of the tube. Further development of the cæcum to form the adult caput coli in these cases leads to the unequal and exaggerated expansion of the ventral and lateral walls of the pouch, as compared with the fixed and adherent dorsal wall. The former are distended and pushed downwards, producing a relative recession of the root of the appendix upward and to the left, until it comes into relation with, or even under cover of, the ileo-colic junction and of the terminal ileal coil entering the colon at this point.

The resulting characteristic adult position of the appendix in these cases is as follows:

The termination of the cæcum proper, and the root of the appendix are under cover of the terminal ileum and frequently adherent to the parietal peritoneum of the iliac fossa (Fig. 555). The distal portion of the appendix remains free, either hanging down and in over the brim of the pelvis (Fig. 542), or turned upwards and to the left and coiled in several turns (Figs. 504, 555 and 556).

FIG. 555.—Human fœtus at term. Ileo-colic junction and cæcum; dorsal view. The area of peritoneal adhesion is seen to involve the dorsal aspect of the cæcum as far as the root of the appendix. (Columbia University Museum, No. 1549.)

FIG. 556.—Human infant. Ileo-colic junction and cæcum, with extensive adhesion to parietal peritoneum. (Columbia University Museum, No. 301.)

Finally the *erect vertical retro-cæcal* position of the appendix presents several important variations in the disposition of the peritoneal investment. In Fig. 503, taken from an embryo of 7.6 cm. vertex-coccygeal length, the early complete recession of the retro-cæcal ileal convolutions has probably permitted an early apposition and adhesion of the beginning of the colon to the dorsal prerenal parietal peritoneum. The subsequent descent into the iliac fossa produces a bend in the ventral wall of the colic tube, with a marked convexity directed downwards and forwards, the apex of the bend situated at or near the level of the ileo-colic junction, while the dorsal colic wall is held by the adhesion to the parietal peritoneum, thus giving a backward inclination to the entire cæcum and appendix. During the subsequent descent of the cæcum proper this bend in the colon is gradually diminished and the tube becomes straightened but the apex of the cæcum remains turned back and the appendix is placed in a more or less vertical erect position behind cæcum and ascending colon.

FIG. 557.—Human adult. Ileo-colic junction and cæcum; ventral view. (Columbia University Museum, No. 1612.)

FIG. 558.—Same preparation as Fig. 557; dorsal view. The appendix, erected vertically between cæcum and colon, is completely imbedded in connective tissue.

As regards the disposition of the peritoneal membrane in this type of appendix the following conditions are to be noted:

(*a*) (Schema,Fig. 552.)—The apex of the cæcum and the entire appendix are extraperitoneal, imbedded in the loose connective tissue which occupies the area of serous obliteration. The line of peritoneal reflection from the dorsal wall of the secondary caput coli to the parietal peritoneum of the right iliac fossa is placed transversely below the true apex of the fœtal cæcum and the root of the appendix. The latter tube, imbedded in connective tissue, passes vertically upwards behind the ascending colon, its tip frequently reaching the ventral surface of the right kidney. A well-marked example of this arrangement in the adult is shown in Figs. 557 and 558 (ventral and dorsal view, with peritoneal reflection and vertical retro-colic appendix).

(*b*) (Schema, Fig. 553.)—In other cases, with the same position of the appendix, the entire cæcum and greater part of the ascending colon remains free. The vertically erected appendix is closely attached to the dorsal surface of the ascending colon, included within the serous investment of the large intestine. The adhesion of the latter is confined to a limited area near the hepatic flexure. Consequently cæcum and greater part of ascending colon can be turned up, away from the parietal peritoneum of the iliac fossa, and the dorsal surface of the appendix shows the free serous covering of the adjacent large intestine.

We may assume that this type of the peritoneal relations of the appendix is produced in one of two ways:

1. Either the retro-colic appendix has become early attached to the adjacent large intestine, whose dorsal surface in large part remains free, or

2. The arrangement of the peritoneum indicated in schema, Fig. 552, may be subsequently changed into that shown in schema, Fig. 553, by a continued downward displacement of the cæcum, producing a secondary serous investment of the dorsal surface of appendix and part of ascending colon.

Examples of this type are found both in infantile and adult subjects.

In Fig. 538, taken from an infant three years of age, the cæcum is lifted up to show the vertical position of the appendix behind the cæcum and ascending colon, the dorsal surface of the large intestine retaining its free serous covering. Another illustration of this arrangement in a juvenile subject is shown in Fig. 529. The same condition in the adult subject is illustrated in Figs. 539 and 540.

FIG. 559.—Human infant. Ileo-colic junction and cæcum; dorsal view. Retro-colic appendix, adherent to the free dorsal serous surface of the large intestine, with intermediate extraperitoneal segment. (Columbia University Museum, No. 1638.)

(*c*) (Schema, Fig. 554.)—Occasionally, with the appendix erected vertically behind the ascending colon, the apex of the cæcum and the proximal portion of the appendix are invested by peritoneum for a short distance and the tip of the appendix likewise obtains a free serous investment, while the intermediate greater portion of the appendix and the corresponding segment of the dorsal surface of the ascending colon are extraperitoneal, adherent to the abdominal parietes. Examples of this peritoneal relation of the appendix in an infant are shown in Figs. 559 and 560, while Fig. 509 represents the same arrangement in an adult specimen. The condition is produced from the arrangement of schema, Fig. 554, by secondary adhesion and obliteration of the serous surfaces over the intermediate portion of the retroverted appendix and the adjacent dorsal surface of the ascending colon.

FIG. 560.—Human adult. Ileo-colic junction and cæcum; dorsal view. Appendix with intermediate non-peritoneal segment, while the proximal portion and the tip are covered by serous investment. (Columbia University Museum, No. 1615.)

C. ILEO-CÆCAL FOLDS AND FOSSÆ.

Certain peritoneal folds, either mesenteric in character, *i. e.*, containing blood vessels, or non-vascular, pass between the terminal ileum and the cæcum and appendix, modifying in some instances very markedly the position and peritoneal relations of the structures.

In considering the influence which these vascular mesenteric and non-vascular serous folds exert in producing further changes in the shape, position and relations of the human appendix it is necessary to remember that in the early embryonal stages these bands and folds of the peritoneum appear only slightly marked, but that they gain their importance and influence on the final adult configuration of the cæcal pouch and appendix in the course of the further development of these structures.

For this reason the comparative study of the corresponding parts in other vertebrates, especially in certain mammalia, is of the utmost value, if we seek to explain and understand the derivation, significance and typical arrangement of these folds. We have seen that the cæcum as found in the large majority of mammalian forms is equivalent to the cæcum and appendix of the human subject and anthropoid apes; that in other words the vermiform appendix represents the distal segment of a cæcal pouch, originally uniform in caliber, which has remained undeveloped, while the proximal portion has progressed evenly with the general development of the alimentary canal to form the cæcum proper. We have seen that this tendency to retain the distal portion of the pouch in a rudimentary condition, *i. e.*, the production of an appendage to the cæcum proper, is encountered in several of the lower forms, as certain Marsupials, Carnivores, Ungulates and Lemurs. The morphology of the ileo-cæcal folds is hence best understood by considering these structures as they appear in connection with the various cæcal types presented by the lower mammalia. Their arrangement and significance can here be readily made out. On the other hand, in studying these structures in the human appendix we are following lines which are already becoming indistinct on account of the rudimentary character of the organ, which we must regard as undergoing an exceedingly slow process of reduction, with a view to its ultimate elimination from the body. We have seen that the structural uncertainty impressed on cæcum and appendix by this evolutionary influence finds its expression in the wide range of variation in size and arrangement which these parts present. Necessarily, of course, this tendency to variation is shared, and even exhibited to a more marked degree, by what we can term the accessory structures connected with cæcum and appendix, viz., the mesenteric vascular and non-vascular serous folds passing to them from the ileum.

We can most profitably begin our consideration of these folds in a form in which they are preserved in their entire and original development, and then successively trace the changes leading up to the normal disposition in the human subject. Such a type is presented by the cæcum of *Ateles ater*, the black-handed spider monkey (Figs. 444 and 445). The cæcum of this animal presents a uniform crescentic curve, with the concavity directed upward and to the left, and the gradual diminution in the caliber of the pouch, from the ileo-colic junction to the apex, denotes the tendency to retain the distal segment in a rudimentary condition, foreshadowing the eventual formation of a vermiform appendix.

In the ventral view, with the terminal ileum lifted up, the following arrangement of folds passing between ileum and cæcum is noted (Figs. 444 and 445).

(*a*) *Vascular Mesenteric Folds.*—The peritoneal vascular folds, carrying the blood vessels to supply the cæcum, are two in number, a ventral (1) and dorsal (3). They are of nearly equal size and extent, passing from the ventral and dorsal aspect of the ileo-colic junction nearly to the apex of the cæcum. Each contains a branch of the ileo-colic artery, which forks in the ileo-colic mesentery, in the angle between ileum and large intestine. The ventral branch continues in the ventral mesenteric fold (Fig. 445) downward across the ventral surface of the ileo-colic junction to supply the ventral part of the cæcum, while the dorsal branch

138

descends behind the ileo-colic junction, preserving a similar course in the dorsal mesenteric fold. The dorsal arterial branch is somewhat larger than the ventral and its distribution extends a little further down to the actual apex of the cæcum.

FIG. 561.—Human adult ileum with Meckel's diverticulum. Ileo-diverticular serous fold and persistent omphalo-mesenteric artery. (Columbia University Museum, No. 1803.)

(b)*Non-vascular Ileo-cæcal Serous Reduplication.*—Between the two vascular mesenteric folds a third serous reduplication, carrying no blood vessels, is found passing between the ileum and cæcum. This fold begins, in the preparation from which the figure is taken, on the ileum opposite the attached mesenteric border, 2.7 cm. from the ileo-colic junction, and passes for exactly the same distance down on the adjacent left concave surface of the cæcum. It is placed a little nearer to the dorsal than to the ventral vascular fold, so that it passes, if the distance between the two vascular folds on the cæcum be divided into three parts, at the junction of the dorsal third with the ventral two thirds. The production of this intermediate non-vascular ileo-cæcal reduplication, which is of very constant occurrence in the mammalian series, is to be led back to the development of the cæcum. When the pouch protrudes from the smooth surface of the embryonic intestine opposite the mesenteric border, it extends backward along the future small intestine and lifts off the serous investment of the gut in the form of a small peritoneal plate filling the interval between itself and the adjacent ileum. A very perfect illustration of this process can be seen in the instance of Meckel's diverticulum shown in Fig. 561. The proximal portion of the diverticulum is here still closely connected to the small intestine along which it extends, both being surrounded by the common visceral peritoneum. The distal part of the diverticulum has separated more completely from the intestine, and in so doing has drawn out the serous investment in the form of the triangular fold which is seen to pass between the free margin of the intestine and the adjacent surface of the pouch. The same process can be followed in its different stages in certain normal mammalian cæcal types.

FIG. 562.—Human adult. Ileum with Meckel's diverticulum, 131.5 cm. from ileo-colic junction; a distinct vascular fold is prolonged from the ileal mesentery to the margin of the diverticulum. (Columbia University Museum, No. 1849.)

In this connection it may be noted that the production of the cæcal vascular folds and their relation to the mesentery is also very perfectly illustrated in some forms of Meckel's diverticulum. Thus in the preparation shown in Fig. 562, a broad triangular serous fold passes from the ileal mesentery to the margin of the diverticulum, carrying the blood vessels which supply the pouch. If the section of the intestine to the left of the figure is regarded as representing the terminal ileum, that to the right the colon, and the diverticulum the cæcal pouch, the formation of the fold and its relation to the mesentery, blood vessels and intestine will correspond closely to the ileo-cæcal vascular folds.

Fig. 350 shows the ileo-colic junction and cæcum of *Halmaturus derbyanus*, the rock kangaroo. The cæcum here extends backwards along the free border of the ileum to which it is closely bound by the common investing visceral peritoneum for the greater part of its extent. In another marsupial form, a small species of opossum from Trinidad (Fig. 349), the cæcum has separated itself more completely from the adjacent small intestine—thus drawing out the peritoneum into a narrow connecting fold. Finally, in the Virginia opossum (Fig. 348), the ileum has attained the usual position at right angles to cæcum and colon. The former pouch is separated from the small intestine by a considerable interval and the angle between the two is filled out by a well-developed triangular serous fold, connecting the free margin of the terminal ileum and the adjacent left border of the cæcum.

This is the "intermediate non-vascular" ileo-cæcal fold.

Passing now from the condition presented by *Ateles*, with three fully developed and distinct ileo-cæcal folds, to the next stage leading up to the normal human arrangement, we find the same illustrated in the cæcum of another new-world monkey, *Mycetes fuscus*, the brown howler monkey, shown in the ventral and dorsal views in Figs. 449 and 450. The ventral vascular fold (Fig. 449, 1) is still well developed, the contained ventral branch of the ileo-colic artery descending over the ventral wall of the ileo-colic junction and cæcum and supplying both. The dorsal vascular fold (Fig. 450, 2), on the other hand, is nearly completely fused with the intermediate non-vascular reduplication (Figs. 449 and 450, 3), the approximation between these structures exhibited by *Ateles* having in *Mycetes* reached the point of actual union, so that the larger dorsal branch of the ileo-cæcal artery descends to the apex of the cæcum in the following manner: The main post-cæcal artery passes over the dorsal surface of the ileo-colic junction included in a short serous fold which corresponds to the dorsal vascular fold of *Ateles*. Beyond the lower border of the ileo-colic junction this fold fuses with the intermediate non-vascular fold, one arterial branch descending along the line of attachment of this fold to the cæcum, the other distributed over the dorsal surface of the pouch.

A third type, also taken from the lower Primates, is presented by the cæcum of a cynomorphous monkey, *Cercopithecus sabæus*, the African green monkey, shown in Fig. 432, in the ventral and left aspect with the terminal ileum lifted up. The cæcum of this animal is comparatively short, somewhat conical, terminating in a blunt apex. The vascular supply is arranged on the same type as in *Ateles* and *Mycetes, i. e.*, a trunk of the ileo-colic artery divides at the ileo-colic notch, one branch descending ventrad, the other dorsad of the ileo-colic junction. The slightly larger size of the dorsal vessel, noted in *Ateles* and *Mycetes*, has been increased in *Cercopithecus* until the ventral artery (1) supplies merely the front of the ileo-colic junction and the upper part of the adjoining ventral wall of the cæcum, while the larger dorsal vessel (2) descends behind the ileo-colic junction, supplying the same and the entire dorsal and apical portions of the cæcum. The relation of these cæcal arteries to the peritoneum is moreover different from that encountered in *Ateles*. In place of running in distinct mesenteric folds, as in the latter species, the vessels pass close to the surface of the intestine, merely covered and partly surrounded by slightly redundant visceral peritoneum containing numerous pads of epiploic fat, which bead the course of the vessels at regular intervals. Between the two arteries the intermediate non-vascular fold (2) is seen, presenting much the same arrangement as in *Ateles* and passing between the left border of the cæcum and the adjacent margin of the ileum, nearer to the dorsal larger than to the ventral smaller cæcal artery.

We have, therefore, in the three types just considered, the following variations in the arrangement of the vascular and non-vascular folds:

a) Ventral and dorsal vascular folds distinct and free. Ventral and dorsal cæcal arteries of nearly equal size.

b) Intermediate non-vascular fold free on both surfaces, placed nearer to the dorsal than to the ventral vascular fold.

Ateles.

a) Ventral vascular fold distinct. Ventral cæcal artery somewhat further reduced in size. Dorsal vascular fold distinct only over the dorsal surface of the ileo-colic junction. At the lower border of the ileo-colic junction the dorsal vascular fold fuses with the intermediate non-vascular fold.

b) Intermediate non-vascular fold free only on ventral surface, the dorsal surface below the ileo-colic junction being fused with the dorsal vascular fold.

Mycetes.

a) Dorsal and ventral vascular folds reduced. Dorsal artery much larger than ventral.

b) Intermediate non-vascular fold well developed, free on both surfaces.

Cercopithecus.

We may judge from this series that the following factors are capable of materially modifying the definite arrangement of the structures:

1. The vascular folds are capable of reduction until the vessels run close to the intestinal surface, merely covered by somewhat redundant peritoneum containing epiploic appendages. (*Cercopithecus.*)

140

2. The dorsal cæcal artery tends to assume in all three forms the greater share in the cæcal vascular supply. This tendency is slightly developed in *Ateles*, becomes more pronounced in *Mycetes*, and is well marked in *Cercopithecus*, in which animal the dorsal vessel nearly replaces the ventral branch, the latter confining itself to the ventral surface of the ileo-colic junction and the adjacent ventral parts of the cæcal wall.

3. The intermediate non-vascular fold is placed nearer to the dorsal larger than to the ventral smaller cæcal artery. This condition, present in both *Ateles* and *Cercopithecus*, foreshadows the fusion of the intermediate and dorsal vascular folds at the lower border of the ileo-colic junction, as seen in *Mycetes*.

4. This fusion of the two folds named in *Mycetes* results in giving different values to the dorsal vascular fold in its proximal and distal segments. The proximal segment descends from the ileo-colic notch behind the ileo-colic junction to its lower border as a distinct fold. Beyond this point its fusion with the distal (cæcal) segment of the intermediate fold rounds out a fossa, the inferior or posterior ileo-cæcal, which is consequently bounded in front by the intermediate vascular fold, behind by the proximal segment of the dorsal vascular fold, to the right side by the inner wall of the cæcum, between the intermediate and dorsal vascular folds, above by the lower border of ileum and ileo-colic junction, and below by the fusion of the two folds.

This pocket or fossa which is the most important and constant of the peritoneal recesses in the neighborhood of the cæcum, opens upward and to the left.

5. A superior or anterior ileo-cæcal fossa, formed in cases of well-developed ventral vascular fold between the same and the ventral wall of the ileo-colic junction, is of small size and shallow.

The cause of the greater development of the dorsal as compared with the ventral cæcal artery is probably to be sought in the adhesion of the colon to the dorsal parietal peritoneum. In *Cercopithecus* the dorsal surface of the ascending colon is adherent to the parietal peritoneum down as far as the iliac region and beginning of the cæcum, whereas in *Mycetes* the entire cæcum, as well as the ascending colon, are free and non-adherent to the abdominal parietes. The influence of this adhesion on the arrangement of the vascular supply of the lower portion of the ascending colon and cæcum appears to be important. Some of the departures from the *Ateles* type presented by *Cercopithecus* become still better developed in the human subject, where the adhesion of the ascending colon and the obliteration of the apposed serous surfaces of ascending mesocolon and parietal peritoneum is normally complete, even if the cæcum remains entirely free, or only adheres to the iliac parietal peritoneum in the proximal part of its dorsal surface. Comparison with forms presenting non-adherent colic and cæcal tubes indicates that the adhesion determines the relative size and arrangement of the ileo-colic vessels.

Thus the partially adherent colon and cæcum of *Cercopithecus* presents, compared with the free tube of *Ateles* and *Mycetes*, a marked reduction of the ventral and a corresponding enlargement of the dorsal cæcal artery. Further progress in the same direction is noted in the human subject where normally the ascending colon and at times the proximal portion of the cæcum are adherent to the dorsal parietal peritoneum.

It appears that in the adhesion of the colic tube to the parietal peritoneum the dorsal ileo-colic vessels find an element favorable to their more complete development and extension, replacing in part or entirely the ventral cæcal artery which becomes limited in distribution to the region of the ileo-colic junction. The adhesion and fixation of the dorsal wall of the intestine seems to afford an advantage to the dorsal vessel, whereas the greater mobility and the alternating conditions of distension and contraction, with variations of intracæcal pressure, depending upon the contents of the pouch, appear to operate unfavorably upon the development of the ventral vessel.

This view is borne out by the conditions observed in the exceptional instances in which in the human subject the ventral artery assumes the large share in the supply of cæcum and appendix (cf. p. 276). In all the cases observed the type of the cæcum indicated delayed or imperfect colic adhesion, and the ascending mesocolon remained partially free.

FIG. 563.—Human; child one year old. Cæcum and ileo-colic junction; ventral view. (Columbia University, Study Collection.)

1. Ventral cæcal artery, surrounded by epiploic appendages.

2. Dorsal vascular fold, forming appendicular mesentery.

3. Intermediate non-vascular fold.

If we now compare the conditions above described for *Ateles,Mycetes, Cercopithecus*with those usually found in man and in the anthropoid apes, we may appreciate the significance of the structures encountered by beginning the investigation with a type in which the derivation of the different parts is still quite evident. Such a condition is presented by the preparation shown in Fig. 563, taken from a child one year of age. Here the descent of the cæcum has evidently been quite rapid and uniform without dorsal adhesion. The cæcum and ascending colon remain free and can still be lifted away from the ventral facies of the right kidney and turned toward the median line to a point somewhat beyond the renal hilus. The cæcum hangs downward vertically and the appendix arises from the funnel-shaped apex of the pouch.

The ventral cæcal branch of the ileo-colic artery is slightly developed, (1) as a small vessel descending in an epiploic fold over the ventral surface of the ileo-colic junction as far as the root of the appendix. The intermediate non-vascular fold (3) is well marked, measuring 2.9 cm. in length, extending from the free border of the terminal ileum to the cæcum and appendix and crossing over the well-developed dorsal vascular fold (2), which descends, as the appendicular mesenterolium, to the tip of the appendix, carrying the dorsal artery. In studying the conditions presented by this specimen, it is not difficult to trace the analogous structures in the cæca of *Cercopithecus, Ateles* and *Mycetes.* The same vascular and non-vascular serous reduplications are found passing between the ileum and cæcum. In accordance with the type presented by *Cercopithecus* the ventral artery is much reduced and runs in a short serous fold loaded with epiploic appendages. The dorsal artery, on the other hand, is well developed and the intermediate non-vascular fold is distinct. In their relative arrangement these folds follow the *Ateles* type. The dorsal vascular fold forms the true mesentery of the appendix, and, although close to and crossed by the intermediate non-vascular reduplication, remains still quite separable and distinct from the same; consequently the lower limit of the usual posterior ileo-cæcal fossa, produced by the fusion of the dorsal vascular and the intermediate non-vascular fold, is absent.

A very perfect illustration of this type of the human ileo-cæcal fold is presented by the preparation of *Gorilla savagei* shown in Fig. 457. The ventral fold and artery appear reduced in this animal. The dorsal vascular fold forms a broad triangular plate of serous membrane carrying the dorsal artery in its free border and extending to the tip of the appendix.

The intermediate non-vascular fold is narrow but distinct, continued for a considerable distance along the ileum, opposite to the attached border, but only for a short extent along the left border of the cæcum below the ileo-colic junction. It crosses the ventral surface of the broad dorsal vascular fold in passing to the cæcum, but remains entirely free and is not adherent to the same.

Consequently here again the dorsal or posterior ileo-cæcal fossa loses its distal limitation. The usual arrangement of the parts, as found in the human subject and derived from the preceding, is well illustrated by another anthropoid ape, *Hylobates hoolock*. Fig. 455 shows the ileo-cæcum of this animal in the ventral view and the homologous parts, as compared with *Gorilla*, are readily recognized. On turning the terminal ileum ventrad and cephalad (Fig. 456), it is, however, seen that the intermediate non-vascular fold does not merely cross the dorsal vascular reduplication, as in *Gorilla*, but that it has begun to adhere to the same at the point of intersection. Consequently a well-marked and clearly limited posterior or dorsal ileo-cæcal fossa is formed, bounded ventrally by the intermediate fold at its accession to the cæcum, dorsally by the proximal part of the dorsal vascular fold, to the right by the left wall of the cæcum, behind by the attachment of the intermediate fold, below by the confluence of the two folds, and above by the lower border of ileum and ileo-colic junction.

The open mouth of the fossa looks to the left. Fig. 464, taken from an adult specimen of the chimpanzee, *Troglodytes niger*, shows the extent of the dorsal vascular fold and of its connection with the mesentery of the terminal ileum.

The intermediate non-vascular fold extends from the ileum downwards along the entire left border of the cæcum to the root of the appendix, fusing with the dorsal vascular fold and rounding out a deep posterior ileo-cæcal fossa.

The typical arrangement, as encountered in the human subject, corresponds closely to the conditions presented by these anthropoid apes.

FIG. 564.—Human adult. Cæcum and ileo-colic junction. (Drawn from preparation in Columbia University, Study Collection.)

1. Dorsal vascular fold at the beginning of the distal free portion, forming the appendicular mesentery.

2. Proximal segment of dorsal vascular fold, fusing with

3. Intermediate non-vascular fold.

4. Rounded edge of union of dorsal vascular and intermediate folds bounding the ileo-cæcal fossa caudad.

5. Point of accession to appendix of proximal branch of appendicular artery derived from posterior ileo-cæcal artery.

In Fig. 564, taken from an adult male human subject, the dorsal surface of the ascending colon and of the ileo-colic junction is adherent to the parietal peritoneum. The distention of the cæcum is nearly uniform, the right sacculation being only slightly larger than the left. The appendix, measuring 18.4 cm. in length, arises from the dorsal surface of the caput coli, 1.7 cm. from the point where the ventral longitudinal muscular band turns around the caudal end of the pouch between the two sacculations, and 3.7 cm. below the caudal margin of the ileo-colic junction.

The dorsal vascular fold (2), forming the broad appendicular mesentery (1), is well developed and free in its distal portion, extending, with gradually diminishing width, to the apex of the appendix. The proximal segment of this fold (between 1 and 2) descends over the dorsal surface of the ileo-colic junction and meets (at 4) the intermediate non-vascular fold (3) which extends between the ileum and cæcum, rounding out a crescentic ridge (4) which bounds the entrance into the posterior ileo-cæcal fossa (between 2 and 3). The influence of the folds and of the blood vessels on the position and curves of the appendix is quite apparent in this preparation.

The dorsal larger branch of the ileo-colic artery, supplying cæcum and appendix, passes over the dorsal surface of the ileo-colic junction (2) where the same, as well as the adjacent dorsal surface of the colon, is adherent to the parietal peritoneum. At the point where the dorsal vascular fold intersects and fuses with the intermediate non-vascular fold (4) the artery divides into a proximal and distal branch. The former proceeds to the cæcum and root of the appendix, reaching this tube at the point marked 5. The latter continues (from 1 on) in the free border of the appendicular mesentery to the beginning of the distal third of the appendix, from which point on the fold extends as a narrow reduplication to the tip of the tube. The segment of the appendix situated between these two main arterial branches is thrown into several coils, the expression of the continued growth between two points relatively fixed by the accession of the two arterial branches. The pathological significance of these bends is apparent when we consider the effect which the kinking of the tube would have on catarrhal and other inflammations accompanied by distension of the appendix.

Typical examples of the posterior ileo-cæcal fossa and of the mutual relationship of the limiting folds are seen in Figs. 565 and 566, both taken from adult human subjects.

FIG. 565.—Human adult, Cæcum and ileo-colic junction with large intermediate non-vascular fold and deep posterior ileo-cæcal fossa. (Columbia University Museum, No. 1546.)

FIG. 566.—Human adult. Ileo-colic junction and cæcum. (Columbia University Museum, No. 1659.)

The significance and mutual relations of the folds seen in the preparations just considered—which illustrate the typical adult human arrangement of the structures—will perhaps be best understood by comparison with an adult cæcum in which the infantile condition, as seen inFig. 563, has become further developed.

FIG. 567.—Human adult. Ileo-colic junction and cæcum; dorsal view. (Drawn from preparation in Columbia University, Study Collection.)

1. Dorsal vascular fold, carrying the distal appendicular branch of the dorsal cæcal artery in the mesentery of the appendix.

2. Proximal branch of the same vessel, turning downward to cæcum and root of appendix.

3. Intermediate non-vascular fold.

Fig. 567 shows the dorsal view of such a preparation. The cæcum is funnel-shaped with the apex, carrying the root of the appendix, turned upward and to the left, the sacculation to the right of the ventral muscular band being somewhat dilated. The appendix—7.2 cm. long—turns sharply upward and to the left, closely applied to the left cæcal sacculation, passes dorsad to the ileo-colic junction and lies in its terminal part under cover of the ileo-colic mesentery. The ventral branch of the ileo-colic artery descends over the ileo-colic junction, supplying the ventral wall of the cæcum. The intermediate non-vascular fold (3) is 3.9 cm. long and entirely free.

The dorsal vascular fold contains the large dorsal branch of the ileo-colic artery, dividing into two main branches. The first of these (1) passes distally in the free edge of the fold to the terminal part of the appendix. The other proximal branch (2) turns downward to the root of the appendix and the adjacent wall of the cæcum, aiding materially in holding the proximal upturned segment of the appendix in contact with the left cæcal sacculation.

The intermediate fold, short in its cæcal attachment, does not meet the dorsal vascular fold at any point, consequently the ileo-cæcal fossa is not limited caudad toward the root of the appendix. The conditions presented by this specimen correspond exactly to those found in the gorilla (Fig. 457) and in the human infantile preparation (Fig. 563).

In comparing Figs. 564 and 567 it will be noticed that the line of fusion between the intermediate fold and the dorsal vascular fold (Fig. 564, 4) corresponds to the point where the dorsal ileo-cæcal artery divides into its proximal and distal branches (Fig. 567, angle between 1 and 2). Fig. 567 shows that the proximal arterial twig, even without fusion with the intermediate fold, suffices to influence to a considerable degree the curves and position of the appendix, inasmuch as it serves to hold the proximal segment of the tube closely applied in the erected position to the surface of the left cæcal sacculation. The intermediate segment of the appendix, between the points of accession of the two arterial branches, is most prone to develop spiral twists and bends, especially when the usual fusion of the two folds takes place and still further fixes the parts, while the distal segment, carrying the narrow crescentic terminal appendicular mesentery, remains free.

FIG. 568.—Human adult. Ileo-colic junction and cæcum. (Drawn from preparation in Columbia University, Study Collection.)

1. Distal and

2. Proximal branch of dorsal ileo-cæcal artery running in dorsal vascular fold.

3. Intermediate non-vascular fold fusing with 2 and forming a narrow caudal limit to the posterior ileo-cæcal fossa.

Finally, in a certain number of cases, an intermediate condition between the types presented by Figs. 564 and 567 is encountered. In Fig. 568 the general arrangement of the parts corresponds pretty accurately to that seen in Fig. 566, but the transition from a completely free intermediate non-vascular fold to one which has begun to fuse with the dorsal vascular fold is evident. The cæcum is bent upward and to the left, the caput coli being formed by the right sacculation. The appendix, 7.8 cm. long, takes a wide ?-shaped curve. The convexity of the proximal curve corresponds to the point where the proximal appendicular artery (2) passes to the tube. The non-vascular intermediate fold (3), measuring 2.2 cm., fuses with the dorsal vascular fold at this point.

The three preparations illustrate serially the share which the peritoneal folds take in the formation of the posterior ileo-cæcal fossa.

In Fig. 566 the failure of the intermediate fold to meet and fuse with the dorsal vascular fold has left the caudal boundary of the fossa (between 2 and 3) incomplete, the ventral and dorsal walls being formed by the folds in question. Fig. 568, in which fusion between the non-vascular and the dorsal vascular folds has commenced, shows the shallow form of the complete fossa under these conditions, while in Fig. 567, with extensive union of the folds, the fossa has correspondingly increased in depth.

FIG. 569.—Human adult. Ileo-colic junction and cæcum. (Columbia University Museum, No. 1610.)

A similar series is shown in Figs. 569, 570 and 571. In Fig. 569, taken from an adult subject, the intermediate non-vascular fold is entirely free, the dorsal branch of the ileo-cæcal artery passes to cæcum and appendix in an area of adhesion between parietal peritoneum and the intestine which includes the dorsal vascular fold. There is consequently no caudal boundary to the ileo-cæcal fossa. Figs. 570 and 571 are both taken from infantile preparations.

FIG. 571.—Human infant. Ileo-colic junction and cæcum. (Columbia University, Study Collection.)

FIG. 570.—Human infant, four days old. Ileo-colic junction and cæcum. (Columbia University Museum, No. 879.)

In Fig. 570 the dorsal vascular and the intermediate folds nearly meet at the root of the appendix. They serve to outline the fossa, which appears completed in Fig. 571 by the actual meeting and fusion of the folds.

The Ileo-cæcal Folds in the Anthropoid Apes.—(1) *Chimpanzee, Troglodytes niger.*

The structures in a juvenile specimen of this animal are shown in Figs. 460 and 461.

The ventral vascular fold (Fig. 460, 3), containing epiploic fat, descends over the ileo-colic junction nearly to the level of the lower ileal margin. The intermediate non-vascular fold (Figs. 460 and 461, 2), derived from the ileum opposite to the mesenteric border, passes to the ventral and left aspects of the cæcum and meets, near the root of the appendix, the dorsal vascular fold (Fig. 461, 3) carrying the dorsal cæcal branch of the ileo-colic artery, which ramifies over the cæcum and supplies the appendix.

The appendix measures 12.3 cm. and presents a terminal hook, slightly dilated.

The appendicular mesentery terminates within the concavity of this hook and measures 1.5 cm. in width at the broadest part, about 4.5 cm. from the root of the appendix.

Figs. 462 and 463 show the cæcum of the adult chimpanzee in the ventral and dorsal view. The ventral vascular fold (Fig. 462, 1) is well developed, heavily fringed with epiploic appendages.

The non-vascular fold is extremely short and tense, fusing with the short appendicular mesentery near the point where in the dorsal view (Fig. 463) the appendix is seen bent at its origin sharply to the right.

Fig. 464, also taken from an adult specimen of the same animal, shows a very well-developed dorsal vascular fold, which fuses with the intermediate fold to limit a distinct ileo-cæcal recess.

The chimpanzee, therefore, agrees closely with the human subject in the arrangement of the folds.

(2) *Orang, Simia satyrus.*

In Figs. 458 and 459 the arrangement of the folds in an adult specimen of the orang is shown.

The ventral cæcal artery (Fig. 458) is well developed, forming with the peritoneal fold and epiploic appendages surrounding it, a sharp sickle-shaped edge which descends over the ventral surface of the ileo-colic junction following the curve of the left cæcal margin, and turning its concavity to the left toward the entering ileum.

The ventral cæcal artery follows the left margin of the cæcum below the ileo-cæcal junction and passes for 0.5 cm. upon the portion of the pouch which turns up behind the terminal ileum.

The dorsal cæcal artery is a vessel of large size, supplying branches to the narrow appendicular mesentery which extends, with many epiploic appendages, to within 9 mm. of the blunt apex of the appendix. 2.5 cm. beyond the first bend in the appendix the fold is narrowed to a fringe not more than 0.75 cm. wide. Up to this point the dorsal vascular fold measures 1.5 cm. in width, and just where it narrows it is joined by the intermediate non-vascular fold (Fig. 459), which forms a membranous band, 3.3 cm. wide in the middle, spread out in the angle between the lower and dorsal surfaces of the ileum and the dorsal surface of the cæcum which turns up behind the ileo-colic junction. Between this fold and the dorsal vascular fold is seen the deep recess of the posterior ileo-cæcal fossa—which by reason of the sharp curve of the cæcum looks not only to the left but also upward and backward.

Direct comparison of the preparations of these two anthropoid apes just described with the conditions found in many adult human cæca shows the close correspondence in the arrangement of these folds and of their influence on the configuration of the parts.

Figs. 572 and 573—taken from an adult human subject—show a cæcum and appendix which almost reproduces that of the chimpanzee illustrated in Figs. 462 and 463 and closely resembles that of the orang.

FIG. 572.—Human adult. Ileo-colic junction and cæcum; ventral view. (Drawn from preparation in Columbia University, Study Collection.)

1. Ventral vascular fold.

FIG. 573.—Dorsal view of the same preparation.

1. Appendix.
2. Intermediate non-vascular fold.

Fig. 572, giving the ventral view, shows, by the course of the ventral longitudinal muscular band, the turn of the cæcum upwards and to the left. The ventral cæcal artery runs in a fold (1) loaded with epiploic appendages.

The non-vascular intermediate fold (Fig. 573, 2) passes to the root of the appendix, joining the proximal segment of the dorsal vascular fold in which the dorsal branch of the ileo-colic artery runs to the tip of the appendix. The distal two thirds of the appendicular mesentery are free.

3. *Gibbon, Hylobates hoolock* (Figs. 455 and 456).—In the gibbon the folds appear well developed. The intermediate and dorsal vascular folds are quite distinct structures, although fusion (Fig. 456) has begun at one point, thus limiting a typical posterior ileo-cæcal fossa.

4. *Gorilla, Gorilla savagei* (Fig. 457).—Finally in the gorilla all three folds appear quite distinct and separate from each other, the dorsal vascular fold being especially well developed.

Unusual and Aberrant Types of Ileo-cæcal Folds and Fossæ.—*(A) Ventral cæcal artery larger than the dorsal, supplying the greater part of the cæcum and the appendix.*

FIG. 574.—Human adult. Cæcum and ileo-colic junction; well-developed ventral vascular fold, carrying appendicular artery. (Columbia University Museum, No. 1613.)

This condition is occasionally encountered. Dr. Martin, in a recent examination of the vascular supply of cæcum and appendix in one hundred subjects, found it to obtain in six instances.

Apparently the dorsal wall of the cæcum and of the proximal segment of the ascending colon remains free in these cases and does not become adherent to the parietal peritoneum. The shape of the pouch, moreover, indicates a free and unimpeded embryonal cæcal descent. The normal relative size of the two vascular folds is reversed. A good example of this variation, in the cæcum of an infant, is seen in Fig. 516. The same arrangement in an adult specimen is seen in Fig. 574.

In the Slow Lemur (*Nycticebus tardigradus*) (Fig. 420) the ventral artery is normally the larger of the two, extending in the ventral fold to the tip of the reduced appendix of the cæcal pouch.

(B) Fusion of ventral vascular fold with the intermediate fold, resulting in the production of a well-defined superior or ventral ileo-cæcal fossa.

FIG. 575.—Human fœtus at term. Ileo-colic junction and cæcum; ventral view. (Columbia University Museum, No. 1715.)

Normally the reduced ventral artery crosses the ileo-colic junction in a slightly developed ventral vascular fold, closely adherent to the intestine, with a very narrow free margin. The superior or ventral ileo-cæcal fossa in these cases is very shallow and confined (Fig. 574) to the ventral surface of the ileo-colic junction. Occasionally the fold is better developed and fuses with the intermediate non-vascular fold, producing a fossa of greater extent, which is bounded dorsad by the ileum, ventrad and cephalad by the ventral fold, caudad by the fusion of this fold with the intermediate reduplication, and to the right by the left wall of the cæcum. Figs. 576,577, 578 and 579 show this aberrant disposition of the structures in a series of adult human cæca.

FIG. 576.—Human adult. Ileo-colic junction and cæcum; ventral appendicular artery and ileo-cæcal fossa. (Columbia University Museum, No. 1614.)

FIG. 577.—Human adult. Ileo-colic junction and cæcum; ventral appendicular artery and ileo-cæcal fossa. (Columbia University Museum, No. 1657.)

FIG. 578.—Human adult. Ileo-colic junction and cæcum; ventral appendicular artery and ileo-cæcal fossa. (Columbia University Museum, No. 1856.)

FIG. 579.—Human adult. Ileo-colic junction and cæcum; ventral appendicular artery and ileo-cæcal fossa. (Columbia University Museum, Study Collection.)

A corresponding arrangement is noted in the preparation of the cæcum of *Cercopithecus campbellii* (Fig. 433). The large intermediate fold is joined by the ventral vascular fold, thus defining the lower boundary of ventral ileo-cæcal fossa.

(*C*) *Union of both vascular folds with the intermediate non-vascular fold.*

FIG. 580.—Human infant. Ileo-colic junction and cæcum; fusion of ventral and dorsal vascular folds, with intermediate fold. (Columbia University Museum, No. 1663.)

I have encountered one instance of this arrangement in an infant, whose cæcum and ileo-colic junction is shown in Fig. 580. Both the ventral and dorsal arteries in this case were equally developed, and shared equally in the supply of cæcum and appendix. Both vascular folds fused with the intermediate fold, thus producing two typical ileo-cæcal fossæ, one ventral, the other dorsal.

(*D*) *Abnormal positions of the appendix due to variations in the arrangement and tension of the intermediate fold.*

Fig. 510 shows a fœtal cæcum in the ventral view. The ventral vascular fold (3) is well developed. The non-vascular fold is short, arising from the ventral surface of the ileum, instead of from the free border of the intestine opposite to the mesenteric attachment. It fuses with the ventral vascular fold a short distance below the ileo-colic junction, thus limiting a small ventral ileo-cæcal fossa. The dorsal cæcal artery in this specimen was large, but the fold carrying it extremely narrow.

The preparation illustrates the type resulting from the reduction in size and extent of the non-vascular and mesenteric folds. The intermediate fold is reduced to a short and narrow band. Compared with the usual infantile type the cæcum lacks the characteristic turn upwards and to the left, possibly in consequence of the slight traction caused by the rudimentary intermediate fold. The pouch occupies a nearly vertical pendent position, which the appendix, arising from the lowest point of the cæcal funnel, shares. The appendix is not drawn into the retro-ileal position by the dorsal vascular fold, which is much reduced.

In Fig. 511, representing the cæcum and appendix of a fœtus at term, the effect of the tense non-vascular intermediate fold (2) is seen in the sharp turn to the left which it imparts to the nearly transversely directed funnel-shaped cæcum. The appendix (1) is coiled spirally for 1¾ turns behind the ileo-colic junction, with the tip directed upward behind the mesentery of the terminal ileum. The non-vascular intermediate fold (2) extends to the rest of the appendix. It appears short in its cæcal attachment, on account of the turn of the cæcum backwards and to the left and the close connection between the adjacent margins of the ileum and cæcum.

FIG. 581.—Human fœtus at term. Ileo-colic junction and cæcum. (Columbia University, Study Collection.)

1. Appendix, terminal portion turned ventrad of ileo-colic junction.

2. Intermediate non-vascular fold.

FIG. 582.—Human infant. Ileo-colic junction and cæcum; ventral position of appendix. (Columbia University Museum, No. 693.)

In Fig. 581—a fœtal preparation at term—the cæcum is turned to the left, below and behind the terminal ileum. The non-vascular fold (2) is well developed as regards *length* of *ileal*attachment, but is very narrow and tense, passing between ileum and the proximal curve of the cæcum behind the ileo-colic junction, where it merges with the dorsal vascular fold. The appendix takes a sudden turn caudad at this point and then continues up *ventrad* to the ileo-colic junction, the proximal portion being kept firmly in contact with the dorsal and caudal circumference of the ileum by the tension of the non-vascular band. It is quite evident that this peculiar turn of the appendix is directly due to the confining influence of the non-vascular band—which passes from its ileal attachment almost directly dorsad to the point of fusion with the dorsal vascular fold, causing the sharp downward and forward turn of the proximal segment of the appendix. Similar cases with ventral position of the appendix are shown in Figs. 545 and 582.

FOOTNOTES:

1In the embryos of reptiles, birds and mammals folds of the somatopleure arise externally to the constricting furrows by means of which the embryo is gradually separated from the yolk-sac, with the resulting formation of the intestinal and abdominal walls. These folds, situated at the head, tail and on the sides, grow upwards and finally meet and unite to form a membranous sac called the *amnion*. Hence these higher vertebrates (reptiles, birds and mammals) are called *Amniota*, in contradistinction to fishes and amphibia who have no amnion and are hence known as *Anamnia*.

2The student should not be confused by the fact that a considerable portion of the pancreatic gland in the cat will be found included between the layers of the great omentum, extending over to the left side of the abdomen. This circumstance will be found of importance in studying the development of the dorsal mesogastrium and of the structures connected with it. For the present attention should only be given to the right extremity or head of the pancreas, situated close to the duodenum and included between the layers of the mesoduodenum.

3For full details of the anatomical and pathological conditions involved consult B. G. A. Moynihan "On Retro-peritoneal Hernia"—London, 1899.

4Iankelowitz, Arch. f. Mikr. Anat., Bd. 46, 1895.

5*Iguana tuberculata*, one of the large lizards native of South America. This animal forms an excellent object for the comparative study of the visceral and vascular anatomy of the abdomen. It possesses a well-differentiated intestinal tract, several coils of small intestine, a well-marked cæcum and large intestine. The examination of this or a similar reptilian form is to be highly recommended. Iguana is easily obtained in any of our large cities, as a considerable number of these animals are annually imported from Mexico and the South American states.

6I am indebted to Dr. J. A. Blake, former Assistant Demonstrator of Anatomy at Columbia University, for the valuable suggestion which led to the preparation ofFigs. 276, 277 and 278 together with the correlated text.

7It should be remembered that in the final adult arrangement of the abdominal viscera the liver shifts relatively backwards, so that the diaphragmatic attachment, originally directed cephalad, now looks dorsad and forms part of the dorsal or "posterior" surface of the adult organ. The original ventral surface looks cephalad, as well as ventrad, forming the convex surface which in the adult rests in contact with the abdominal wall and diaphragmatic vault, while the surface originally directed dorsad toward the stomach finally in large part has an inclination caudad forming the "inferior" surface of human anatomy.

8Flower and Lyddecker, "Mammals, Living and Extinct," p. 209.

9A. v. Haller, Elements physiologiæ, Tom. 7, Liber 24, Sect. 3.

10Fr. Arnold, Handbuch der Anat. d. Menschen. 1847. II. Bd., cloth, p. 84.

11E. Zuckerkandl, "Ueber die Obliteration des Darmfortsatzes beim Menschen." Anat. Hefte XI. (Bd. IV., Heft 1), 1894, p. 107.

12N. Y. Med. Journal, Vol. LXIX., No. 14, p. 508.

13Cf. Quain.

www.ingramcontent.com/pod-product-compliance
Lightning Source LLC
Chambersburg PA
CBHW07085818 0526
45168CB00005B/1871